How to Measure & Change Your Body's Age

GROWING YOUNGER

Dr. Robert F. Morgan
with Jane Wilson
Morgan Foundation Publishers

Copyright © 2000, 2004 Robert F. Morgan

All Rights Reserved. No part of this book may be copied or reproduced, stored in a retrieval system, or transmitted in any form, or by any means mechanical, electronic, photocopying, recording or otherwise, without the prior written permission of the publisher:
305 Mission Serra Terrace, Chico, CA 95926 USA
Fax (815) 550-4456 Phone (530) 892-2131
email: morganfoundtion@earthlink.net
Web page: http://www.morganfoundationpublishers.com

Library of Congress Cataloging in Publication Date

Morgan, Robert F.
   Growing Younger

      Bibliography: p.
      Includes index.
      1. Longevity.   2. Aging.   3. Health.
       I. Wilson, Jane, 1953-   II. Title.
QP85.M58   613   82-42854

ISBN 1-885679-09-2

Second Printing

Printed in the United States of America by:
Amazing Experiences Press
1908 Keswick Lane
Concord, CA 94518
925-825-6060

          10 9 8 7 6 5 4 3 2 1

For Becky

I dedicate this book to all my family, but especially Angel Kwan-Yin Morgan and Cinnamon Morgan, daughters who, during the writing of the manuscript, kept me young better than any megavitamin could. They and my wife Becky Owl Morgan have so enriched my life that its extension could only be delightful.
—*R.M.*

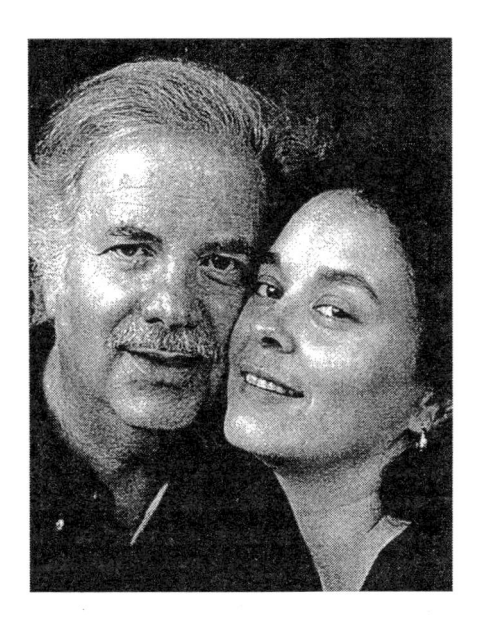

With a special dedication to John Glenn whose 1998 voyage rediscovered our future.

CONTENTS

Acknowledgments vii
Introduction xi

1. Looking at the Past:
   Death as the Yardstick 1

2. Looking at the Family Album:
   Body Age Testing 9

3. Looking at Hypnosis:
   The Elkind Effect 25

4. Looking in the Mirror:
   Self Programming 39

5. Looking at Nutrition:
   Eating and Aging 53

6. Looking at the Thermometer:
   Metabolic Aging 69

7. Looking Outside Ourselves:
   Altitude, Anthropology and Attitude 79

8. Looking Beyond Preconceptions:
   The Human Potentials Movement and Transpersonal Aging 111

9. Looking at Each Other:
   Work, Sex, Love and Purpose 123

10. Looking at the Clock:
    Time and Aging 131

11. Looking at Mistakes:
    Iatrogenic Hazards and Aging 153

12. Looking at the Future:
13. The Phoenix Lodge 171

    Bibliography 175

    Test Manual for the
    Adult Growth Examination 217

    Bibliography 255

    Index 265

ACKNOWLEDGMENTS

FIRST, I gratefully wish to acknowledge Jane Wilson's energy, commitment, and reportorial ability, which lent a new dimension to our work.

If I put my debts in chronological order (and why not, given the present topic?), I would look back to the thorough and catalytic lectures given by the late Stanley C. Ratner, psychologist at Michigan State University. One of these lectures set off a chain of thinking that eventually led to the development of the ADULT GROWTH EXAMINATION body test. Subsequent conversations with Michigan State University professors Paul Bakan, Abram Barch, S. Howard Bartley, M. Ray Denny, Robert L. Green, John King, James Mullin and Hans Toch were also of considerable benefit.

My work on the causes and treatment of senile psychosis was considerably enriched by Bertram Karon (also of MSU), Howard Gudeman and Robert Hunt of Hawaii State Hospital Among the many who have contributed to my education in experimental or clinical areas, I would like to thank Roberto Moulun, George Flanagan, David Tillim, Thomas Toy, Stanley Fevens, David Cheek, Eugene Turrell, Sanford Harris, Richard Weiser, Ed Haupt, Patricia Norman, S. Don Schultz, Sean Abell, Ben Camo, Akasha Morgan, Luke Morgan, Erik Tong and Family, Gene T. Orro, and Nicholas Cummings. I remain impressed by the continued youth, vitality and generosity of co-searchers such as Leonard Elkind, Larry Casler, Sula Benet and the many others whose work, while helping to shape this book, continues to shape the future of both applied and basic gerontology.

I am grateful to the many pioneers who have contributed either directly or indirectly to the growth of the new field of applied gerontology: the study of human aging and its attendant problems. To Sir

Growing Younger

Francis Galton and Hermann von Helmholtz in the nineteenth century as well as to contemporary leaders and innovators such as James and Betty Birren, William Forbes, Alice Dawson, Warren Baller, Alexander Leaf, Barnett Rosenberg, Clive McCay, Phil Zimbardo, Milton Erickson, Linn Cooper, K. Warner Schaie, Alex Comfort, Lissy Jarvik, Bernard Strehler, Hans Selye, Frederick LeBoyer, Tom Veiny, Nathan Pritikin, Michael Lesser, I.M. Murray, C.L. Rose, Erdman Palmore, H. LeCompte, Den-ham Harman, and, particularly Ward Dean, we owe a debt for bringing about the birth and development of a fresh approach toward the understanding and resolution of the problems we call "aging."

Special thanks are due to body-age task force team members Mary Close, Sheila Connolly, Charlotte Gibson, Airi Koivula, Wayne Oake, Joy Spears, and particularly, Tom Malcomson. His work-in-progress on the effects of early retirement on body age should open new vistas. I also look to the work of signal processing engineer N.H. Morgan and his group for future breakthroughs. The courage of Marg Meston and "Marlene," the creativity of Alan Edmonds and the expertise of Victor Rausch must be acknowledged as well, as their contributions have been central to the vitality of this book.

Jon Herron's careful and effective editing and printing also deserve special recognition.

Finally, I would like to acknowledge all those, readers or researchers, whose imagination is not so limited as to ask why anyone would wish to extend a youthful life.

—ROBERT F. MORGAN

Acknowledgments

I would like to thank Dr. Robert Morgan for affording me the chance to explore, in depth and with fresh insight, the complex and lifelong process of aging. When I first entered the AGE laboratory at Wilfrid Laurier University I was 27 years old. I emerged with a body age of 19, the lowest score possible with Dr. Morgan's test. I must admit that adolescence is much better the second time around.

I also would like to mention my grandparents, Lydia and Archie Wills and Isabell Wilson, all well into their ninth decade. Thank you for your genes and for the luster and vitality you have passed on to my generation.

—JANE WILSON

INTRODUCTION

Society is always taken by surprise by any new example of common sense.
—RALPH WALDO EMERSON

ONE OF MY earliest clinical responsibilities was to provide psychotherapy for older adult patients who had been labeled senile. They showed signs of being withdrawn, frightened and confused, and as part of the treatment process I encouraged them to develop individual strategies for confronting the threat of death. This was not easily done; it often took many months of careful preparation. When the time came for sharing these strategies I, as the therapist, was not excluded from the task.

Many of the group members thought they would meet death on spiritual grounds by going back to their church and becoming more devout in their beliefs; one person took up meditation, another turned to death-related art, and a few others adopted the pantheistic philosophy that there was life in all things and that death was just a change of state. I was among those who chose to fight. Long after the senile behavior had faded from our group, we kept in touch with each other to check our progress. In a way, this book is my progress report. If there is to be a fight, I would like to be in the front lines with good measures to keep score.

Gerontology is the study of aging; in itself it is an old science. However, in the last fifty years impressive research has been accumulated and continues to grow. Practitioners in the field, operating under various career labels, rise up daily against the many problems of their aging clients.

As the number of post-retirement citizens climbs in proportion to the total population, and more importantly, as aging citizens become more assertive and better organized, everyone, including government, has begun to pay more attention to aging. As a result, gerontology has attained a higher priority for funding, with some of the money going to basic researchers likely to be unconnected to the survival problems of people. Other funds go to field workers also likely to be unconnected to the researchers, and left to rely on guesswork and guts for their solutions. But the information the researchers come up with is potentially extremely important for the field workers whose questions would help the researchers continue their work effectively. A bridge is needed, and I call that bridge *applied gerontology,* the application of scientifically validated research to resolve the problems of human aging.

Applied gerontology attempts to close the gap between discovery and practical application. Just as gerontology and geriatrics before it, it will ultimately develop into its own discipline. In the meantime, it is interdisciplinary, in that it blends the life and natural sciences with the behavioral and social sciences. While applied gerontologists are intensely interested in the roles of "senior citizens," they view the entire lifespan as something warranting change, from childhood—perhaps even the pre-natal period—through the key transition stages of life. Practitioners may specialize in problems of the middle years, a time when motivation and opportunity are high, but no age group should be excluded. Although old people are of great value to our society, old age is not. By defining the aging 'process in terms of a measurable decline in body functions, I do not wish to downplay the benefits of accumulated experience. I only acknowledge that the pattern of aging we now consider normal runs downhill, and at varying rates. I have chosen to measure those things that affect this process.

Aging may be defined as a series of disadvantaging events that normally occur in our bodies over time. These events gradually reduce our ability to adapt to our surroundings in such a way that they increase the probability of death. The less efficient our bodies become, the more chances we have of dying sooner.

A disease that is not normal for a species in its ordinary lifespan, such as a plague or flu epidemic, would not be considered as aging. On the other hand, some "normal" aging processes are identified as health problems and can be effectively treated as such—for example, high blood pressure and problems related to hearing and vision. Note also that something can be" normal" but need not be inevitable. In many cultures, poverty, whether monetary

Introduction

or intellectual, is characteristic, yet I believe it can be combated.

Aging processes, in some cases, change so reliably with each year of life that by measuring them we can accurately predict the passage of years, much like the rings in a tree trunk that denote the age of the tree. By simple observation, it is fairly easy for people to distinguish a young adult from an old one. Such observation will often be accurate to the nearest decade, but for a scientific study of aging, we need a more reliable system of measurement. By using standardized body-age testing methods we can predict the exact body age. In most cases, it will be accurate within one to five years.

The "growing old" processes are often rooted in childhood, where they were masked by the dynamic "growing up" processes of youth. Their nature is cellular, metabolic, behavioral, organic and molecular. Yet as we age, not everything that occurs is negative. For example, increased experience and the occasional wisdom that stems from it are of definite advantage to the older adult. Thus I distinguish between *aging* and *growth*. By conquering aging we could remove the negative properties that separate the old from the young, without negating the genuine advantages of accumulated experience.

There does exist, however, a general resistance to the idea that the aging process can or should be influenced in the same way that disease can and should be prevented. In some scientific circles, these optimistic goals are regarded as extreme. It has long been easier to get support for programs to ease the symptoms of aging rather than for those that could effect a cure; for programs that aid in the adjustment to life's early end rather than extend life. I have heard academics with impeccable credentials say that "aging cannot be slowed" or "your success in slowing it is neither ethical nor useful." Usually both statements, although contradictory, come from the same individual.

In my opinion, age can be effectively measured and treated. We may regard chronological age—the passage of time since birth—as one way to measure it. Or we can measure body age, social age (maturation) and self-concept age (how old you feel), which depend on what happens to us in the course of our lives. It is this non-calendar aging that is the focus of my work.

Body age is based on the physical aspect whereas social age is behavioral. Self-concept age refers to the normal human process of

Growing Younger

stabilizing, consciously or unconsciously, at a specific year in one's life. It can often be determined through hypnosis if not from observing obvious behavior. Test your memory—at five years of age you undoubtedly were well aware of how different you were from your four-year-old self. Yet, as the years went by, the differences marking one year from the next seemed to diminish until, perhaps one year in your mid-20s, you felt no older than in the previous year. Even the occasional traumatic move from one decade to the next (for example, a 40th birthday) only seemed to change this concept on the surface. Many adults who have lived for more than 80 years have reported to me the recurring shock when they looked in the mirror in the morning and wondered, "Who is this old face looking at my young self?" At such times, their 20-year-old self-concept age was in conflict with their 80-year-old body age.

If you are in your twenties, try imagining yourself waking up after a long sleep (perhaps following an incredible party), walking to the mirror and seeing an 80-year-old version of yourself looking back at you. After the initial shock you might feel depressed at the loss of 60 years to your Rip Van Winkle snooze. Since time is characteristically experienced as passing more quickly with every decade of life, it is understandable that many 80-year-olds often wonder where the last 60 years have gone.

However, something can be done about this. Experienced time can be slowed, expanded and used more productively. Body aging can be slowed, even halted for a while. Yet, with our current technology it is easier to keep a 20-year-old young through prevention than to bring an 80-year-old back to the age of 20 through correction. This book therefore will be of greatest benefit to adults in the 19 to 71-plus age range. It is not a book about the "aged" or "old age"; it is for you and the people you care for, to help you and them in your attempts to grow without growing old.

I am a psychologist. Therefore my work takes a psychological perspective of aging; the focus is on the success and the survival of the individual. This bias has been reduced, to some extent, by the inclusion in this book of work from disciplines as diverse as anthropology and biophysics.

Aging, like all other life processes, is never a reflection of only one influence. There are many useful ways of viewing it, many rea-

Introduction

sons for its occurrence, and many ways to deal with it effectively. No single cause of or cure for aging will likely be found. At present it is accelerated by so many aspects of our lives that countering any one of dozens of disadvantages—pollution, smoking, poor nutrition—must lead to improved health and longevity. If we were to use everything science has taught us to date, I feel that 140 years would be a reasonable expectation for the human life span—a vigorous, youthful 140 years at that. Spectacular breakthroughs in genetics and organ regeneration would take us even farther. In the meantime; although we are awash in the present sad reality of 78 years of average life expectancy, I believe we can show good results by using a variety of anti-aging treatments.

I share the bias for prevention over treatment. Aging often has a pediatric history because we tend to reproduce and build on our' past experiences biologically as well as psychologically. Productive change is always possible but it becomes less probable with every passing year.

I view the mind as a dimension of the body rooted in the nervous system, not as something separate from the body. Therefore, the mind is of great importance to the complete study of aging. Historically, psychologists have moved away from the analysis of the elements of thought and redefined themselves as explorers of behavior. But contemporary psychology is taking a long, fresh look at consciousness as an area worthy of exploration after all. The "mind" dimension of the body represents one of our most potent treatment areas for affecting aging, or "growing younger."

How can we know which explanations for aging are correct? How do we find our way through the maze of blind alleys and useful paths? I have chosen, whenever feasible, to use the scientific method as the "way of knowing." Collecting data systematically leads to a theory with predictions that can be tested, resulting in turn in an improved theory. If we can elevate the scientific method above faith, mysticism and force of authority then, ironically, we may find ourselves in the most unusual belief system of all. Honestly practiced, the scientific method is the most immune to conventional wisdom, or "the way the world is supposed to be." In a study of aging, while avoiding mystification and hoax, a few useful theories will emerge. They may have less than total acceptance among the elite of the aca-

Growing Younger

demic community, but they will not be discarded, once the scientific method has suggested them to be of value. I believe there is a communication lag between what we know and what is practiced. Our pool of knowledge on aging is modest, yet even this modest knowledge is too little reflected in our society, in our lifestyles or those of our children.

Readers using this book in conjunction with the proper test equipment can learn important self-monitoring skills to help them study their own aging and find ways to combat it. However, this book alone is insufficient to train fully qualified professionals in the measurement and treatment of adult aging. Obviously, there are limits to the effectiveness of any assessment technique, including those used in this book. Even the most reliable and valid test administered under controlled conditions will be influenced by the skill of the examiner, the varying states of the subject being tested and the utilization of the findings.

Grow we must. But now we can choose to discover some things that accelerate our aging and others that realistically may bring about our growing younger.

~1~
Looking at
THE PAST
Death as the Yardstick

HOW OLD ARE YOU? These four little words usually hit the target like a pair of loaded dice, weighted by the dealer. When you are asked how old you are, the words can wrap themselves around your innermost fears and insecurities. The answer is just a number, an abstract, an everyday vital statistic similar to your height, your address, how many children you have, the number of cars you own or where you went to school. But if the question touches off an involuntary shudder or a deep sigh, followed by drooping spirits, if you become embarrassed or dismayed, take heart—you're not alone! Remember how as a youngster you were never old *enough?* When birthdays were celebrated milestones representing happy rites of passage? Then suddenly, the milestones became a millstone around your neck. You realized that you were older than you thought; older, perhaps, than you wanted to be. "Ah well," you said to yourself, we grow up and we grow old. Our bodies age. That's just the way things are." But is it?

Many people think aging is measured by birth certificates, calendars and revolutions of the earth around the sun. When you look into the mirror at night, you know that you will wake up one day older in the morning. It doesn't matter that you don't feel as though you are getting older, or that you may not look too different as the years roll by.

Career-minded people, at the age of 35, may have the business world at their feet. At 55, having accumulated experience and (maybe) even wealth, new jobs are harder to come by. At 35, a homemaker may be worked off her feet; at 55 she suffers from an

Growing Younger

empty nest. If a 40-year-old man forgets his hat at a party, it is regarded as an oversight; at 75 a sentence of senility may be pronounced.

Such are the foibles of modern humanity. In simpler times the aged were revered. They commanded respect because they embodied wisdom. Unfortunately, in western society aging has become synonymous with old age, with physical deterioration, declining productivity, uselessness, helplessness, loss of station and ultimately, death.

Preying on the vanities and fears of modern men and women, manufacturers are promoting a myriad of anti-aging creams and lotions, diets, clothing and lifestyles. But while they catch our eyes through glitzy advertising campaigns, the most basic anti-aging advice—good nutrition, no smoking, proper exercise and relaxation—continues to be ignored.

People have been looking for the Fountain of Youth for centuries. And why not? It's an admirable quest and a worthwhile adventure into the unknown. "Why," they ask, "can't we grow younger instead of older? Why do some people, by 'force of nature,' age better than others? Why do some live lengty, healthy lives, while others find their bodies succumbing to disease?"

We are only beginning to find out. Most of what we know about aging and longevity is based on research that uses death as the only measuring stick. It is true that death is the end of the aging process, but it is not its only measure.

The termination of life has long obsessed society. We have chosen to deny it, fear it, covet it and count on it. Some of the more philosophical among us say that death is nature's way of telling us to slow down. As far back as the early 1900s, some scientists viewed death as the triumph of the unnecessary disease of aging. A person's death also may be viewed as a kind of permanent sabbatical with some real benefits to those who are left behind. I recall the inadvertent mispronouncement of one university administrator concerning three faculty members destined to return from leave: "Their absence will be sorely missed."

Death makes a poor yardstick to measure aging in adults. Yet, there are some important leads that such information can give us. Vital statistics on current human mortality are available from several

sources, including the World Health Organization, the Metropolitan Life Insurance Company, the National Center for Health Statistics, the United States Public Health Service and the American Heart Association. From their recently published records we can compare people's survival figures on the basis of their chronological age, where they live, their sex, their race and the cause of their demise. In this context, some basic patterns have emerged:
- Men over age 45 whose names are listed in *Who's Who* are likely to live longer than the general population.
- The Number One cause of death is disease of the heart and of the blood vessels.
- Celibacy and lack of companionship lower the age at which you are likely to die.
- Competitive athletics can be as detrimental to your longevity as doing no exercise at all: moderate exercise for fun seems to be the best route to follow.
- A death rate is the percentage of people expected to die at any given age. In the United States, counties with the highest proportion of death rates tend to be those located on the Atlantic or Gulf coasts and at low altitudes, while those with the lowest death rates tend to be at higher elevations. Areas with low death rates also had more residents over 65 than the high death rate counties, so their greater survival was not due to a younger population. Speculation is that people who live at higher altitudes have a greater lung capacity, get more exercise, better preserve their energy, enjoy clean air and water and benefit from living in smaller communities.
- There is some evidence that certain blood types (A, P2, Le) are associated with greater longevity.
- Mortality from lung cancer has increased tremendously since 1950, with the greatest risk now occurring among younger adults. The incidence of chronic bronchitis has doubled since then. Also showing a significant increase are diseases such as cirrhosis of the liver, emphysema and arteriosclerotic heart disease. From 1950 to 1966, lung cancer mortality for men registered a 113% increase; among women it rose 58%. More recent data confirms a continuation of this pattern with increasing number of deaths resulting from cancer, diabetes mellitus, bronchi-

tis, emphysema, asthma, cirrhosis of the liver, suicide and homicide.

The gloomy picture reflected in this last pattern is contrary to the commonly held belief that over the last few decades our lifespan has increased through medical advances. The National Center for Health Statistics confirmed that the average life expectancy from birth is 78 years (80 for females, 74 for males). Yet, in this analysis we saw as the causes of death a continuing increase in cirrhosis of the liver and in homicide. The factor most responsible for the longer average lifespan today seems to be the decrease in infant mortality. But for mature adults the probability of longer survival has not greatly improved. This means, in effect, that nowadays babies have a better chance to live to be adults than adults have to live much past their retirement age. For statisticians who spend their time demonstrating the superiority of our medical technology, these figures can be frustrating.

The turning point came in the 1950s when the negative aspects of our environment equaled medical progress and began to surpass it. In a 1964 analysis, I.M. Moriyama, an American government statistician, announced: "After a longer period of decline, the trend of the crude death rate appears to have leveled off. In the United States, the crude death rate has been more or less stationary during the period 1950-1960. The failure to experience a decline in mortality during this period is unexpected in view of the intensified attack on medical problems in the postwar years ... at no time in the history of the country have conditions appeared so favorable for health progress.

How did he explain it? "Radioactive fall-out, air pollution and other manmade hazards cannot be completely ignored... [but] it is obviously impossible for the death rate to decline indefinitely. At some point in time the mortality rate must level off as it reaches the irreducible minimum."

Invoking an "irreducible minimum" of progress to combat death was typical of the official optimism displayed by the U.S. Public Health Service at the time. If we were making no more progress against mortality, they insisted that it was because we had done everything that could be done. The "manmade hazards" were minimized and the possible dangers of alcohol and tobacco were not

Looking at the Past

even mentioned. Undercutting this point of view were the unhappy results of subsequent years that showed the so-called "golden plateau" giving way to increasing mortality in areas definitely connected to "manmade hazards" including tobacco, drugs, alcohol, suicide and homicide. While we are succeeding in keeping babies safe, we are killing adults in proportionately greater numbers. Cancer, for example, will now kill one in four; one million are treated for it in the United States alone every year and more than one-third of them will die from it. While it is true that the average lifespan has risen from 47 years in 1900 to 78 years in 2000, this is so much a product of infants' greater survival rate that the years remaining to a 55 year old are only a few more on the average than in 1900. If it is true that there have been medical advances, where is the increased mortality coming from? Biochemist Dick Passwater blames malnutrition at all economic levels. The citizens of thirty nations have been identified on the average as enjoying greater life expectancies than we do in North America.

Another factor strongly associated with early mortality is obesity. Biochemical research on rats has shown that under-feeding in youth extends the lifespan of the animals. (Further details in Chapter Five.) Yet, the final phase of life should not be characterized by weight loss. Longest life and lowest disease rates may be associated with low body weight in early and middle life with some modest gain in the end phase. Among rats whose food intake was restricted while they were young, those who weighed the most in old age lived the longest. Could it be pleasure from regaining the forbidden fruit? If we speculate on the basis of such research we might conclude that old age is no time for crash diets. Any attempts to reduce obesity for those over 65 should be under close and responsible medical supervision. For pre-retirement age adults, low body weight seems worth accomplishing, particularly in order to avoid heart attacks. The Metropolitan Life Insurance Company tells us that when adult body weight is 20% above average, mortality increases 31% for men aged 15 to 69, and 32% for women aged 40 to 69 (21% for women aged 15 to 39). The best plan might be to stay thin from childhood on, and move to average weight after 65.

Now that we know that adults should be neither emaciated nor obese, let us better define our terms. Obesity has been commonly

Growing Younger

defined as any weight 20% or more above average. However, the average Canadian or American has become so rotund that a safer goal for the longevity-minded would be to not exceed the average at all. The following example is taken from a Public Health Service survey of 6,672 representative United States citizens. The weights were taken with the subjects stripped to the waist and with their shoes off. Subtract two pounds to obtain nude weight.

The average American woman is *5'2"* tall, weighs 142 pounds, has a waist measuring 30", a chest of 35" and a seat breadth of 14".

The average American man is 5'8" tall, weighs 168 pounds, has a waist measuring 35", a chest of 39" and a seat breadth of 14".

MEN:		WOMEN:	
Height (in.)	Weight (lbs.)	Height (in.)	Weight (lbs.)
73	191	68	150
72	188	67	154
71	181	66	139
70	180	65	142
69	173	64	140
68	165	63	135
67	167	62	133
66	161	61	127
65	156	60	124
64	147	59	118
63	143	58	121
62	139	57	128

(Height and weight including approximately 2 lbs. clothing)

(Seat breadth, by the way, is the distance across the greatest lateral protrusion on each side of the buttocks.)

Similar surveys in Canada and Great Britain have shown American men to be 5 pounds heavier than Canadian men and 19 pounds heavier than British men. American women average 5 pounds more than Canadian women and 14 pounds more than British women. American mortality figures are head and shoulders above Canadian and British ones as well.

What should we weigh? Borrowing again from Public Health

Service figures, let us use the 25- to 34-year-old averages as the weights that we should not exceed. The table on page 6 shows a very conservative estimate.

Based on the vital statistics we so far have accumulated, what predictions can we make about longevity? We have added more than 50 years of life to the 22 years a Roman expected to live before the birth of Christ, yet we may well add another 50 years in the near future. Rand Corporation scientists predicted in 1964 that we would achieve our next 50 years of life by the year 2020. Five years later, scientists from another laboratory advanced the target year to the early 1990s.

On the other hand, we also know that there is a high probability of death occurring in the first three months of residence for anyone committed to the institutions for the aged.

While advice concerning how to live a longer life is probably as old as the history of human speech, mortality research has shown that the following are still the most valid predictors:

—Work satisfaction
—No cigarette smoking
—No cardiovascular disease
—High personal happiness
—Good health and basic physical functioning
—High intelligence
—A positive view of life
—A useful and satisfying role in society
—A sound financial status
—An intact marriage
—Few worries
—Conserving personal energy

—A marriage in which one spouse is younger than the other
—Up to the age of 40, looking young for one's age
—Not being easily aggravated
—Having been raised in a small family
—Continuing work activity after retirement age
—Long-lived parents
—Having been raised by a young mother

Long life depends on a complex combination of physical, social and genetic factors described as "élite status." In other words, happy, satisfied people, with high intelligence, sound finances, well-maintained health and intact marriages may expect to live a good deal longer than their less-intelligent, poorer relations whose health is declining and whose marriages are not intact.

Growing Younger

Using death statistics to compile information on what speeds up or slows down aging has its limitations. In fact, there is more to aging than death and more to living than survival. We need to measure aging long before it threatens our existence.

~2~
Looking at
THE FAMILY ALBUM
Body Age Testing

PEOPLE GROW OLD at different rates. There are 40 year olds with bodies that have aged only 25 years, and *25* year olds with bodies of 40 year olds. Often, simple observation will tell you whether men or women have aged above or below their years. The body and the face reveal signs of good health, fitness, contentment and freedom from the ravages of time and the environment people live in — factors that the age marked on their birth certificates doesn't take into account. If we can determine our physical age and keep track of what happens to our bodies as time progresses, is it not reasonable to assume that we could manage our health and our aging better?

Until recently, no method had been found to evaluate the aging of the human body, except to use death as the ultimate yardstick. Indeed, until now the only way to tally the individual rate of aging was to record the passage of time since birth — a chronology based on the circuits of the earth around the sun — rather than chronicle the obvious changes that take place as we move across time, at our own speed, from birth to death.

Over a period of 15 years, studies have been conducted on about 9,000 people. As a result we have been able to devise a quick and simple test to measure the fitness of one adult body and compare it to that of others born at the same time.

Let's say you are 40 years old. After your annual physical examination your doctor tells you that you have the body of a 25 year old. Kudos are in order, of course, but it is unlikely that your doctor has any concrete basis for making his remark, as he probably hasn't examined enough 25 year olds to know exactly what their bodies *should* be like. The Adult Growth Examination (AGE) can effectively measure three physical features that deteriorate as the body gets older, and they have been found to be representative of the state of the body as measured against time. If you cannot fully accept your doctor's compliment, the 15-minute AGE test can check his estimate.

Accurate description is crucial to any science. However, it becomes mystified and handicapped when descriptions of what *is* are confused with what *must be*. We know that all but the simplest organisms on our planet age reliably but, because aging is a complex response to an equally complex environment, we can change the organism's behavior by changing key parts of that environment. Enough is now known to influence the rate of human aging. In time, the basic nature and existence of the process may be discovered and thereby controlled. If we know the consequences of our actions we can more effectively make a better world to live in and contribute to a better self. Not everyone would choose to extend his or her life, even if there were a guarantee that it would be devoid of senility and endowed with vigor to the last moment. However, those who would *do* have the right to exercise this option. The Adult Growth Examination and the study of aging may be one way to realize this right of personal choice.

First, let me give you a bit of history. As far back as 1856, the German scientist Herman von Helmholtz observed that there were individual differences in the optical physiology of aging. He focused his findings on presbyopia, a form of farsightedness that occurs as people get older, making it difficult for them to see things clearly at close range. Helmholtz noted that people suffering from early progressing presbyopia died earlier than those with late progressing presbyopia. A few decades later, in 1884, the British scientist Sir Francis Galton, after testing more than 9,000 people between the ages of 5 and 80, confirmed that both vision *and* hearing deteriorate with age.

In the early 1930s H. Steinhaus, a European mathematician, followed up on the work of both von Helmholtz and Galton; he began a careful study of 5,000 patients who had complained of eye problems over a long period of time. The results of his investiga-

Looking at the Family Album

tions were published in 1932, based on 1,000 death records. They confirmed a high correlation between presbyopia and early mortality. Steinhaus found middle-age farsightedness to be primarily a predictor of death by heart disease, and so potent an aging characteristic that it was not affected by social class, rural or urban living conditions or sex differences. In 1945, mathematician Felix Bernstein suggested that it was justifiable to use the Steinhaus studies of presbyopia as the basis for indexing physiological aging. Although it was an intelligent and well-founded recommendation, it was generally ignored by the medical community.

However, for the past three decades scientists have become increasingly aware of the need to test body age as the first step toward gathering information about how and why people age the way they do. Numerous tests were formulated, based on sexual functions, vision, strength, blood tests, urine samples, biopsies of gray hairs,* blood pressure and a variety of other variables. Attempts also were made to develop an age test using the abilities of industrial workers as criteria. Among the most valuable contributions in this field was the systematic health measures survey compiled by F.E. Linder and his colleagues at the United States Public Health Service. More interested in health than in aging, the team collected essential data on adults of all ages. After carefully selecting a representative sample of the American people, they published their findings in 1962. After testing nearly 7,000 persons between the ages of 18 and 79 years, the results confirmed the sensitive age indices of near vision, hearing level at high frequency, systolic blood pressure and various other measurements.

My own involvement in body age testing began in 1960, when I heard an engaging and catalytic lecture on general psychology by Professor Stanley C. Ratner at Michigan State University. After reviewing the theory and practice of standardized testing, he went on to discuss a new unit—the physical effects of aging with special emphasis on presbyopia.

The seeds of what was to become the Adult Growth Examination had been planted. I suggested a combination of these two areas,

---
*Recent studies have shown gray hair, white hair and baldness in adults to have little relationship to aging. Loss of hair color seems to be more the result of stress, heredity or dietary deficiency; hair loss may be the result of extra sex hormones.

11

and while working as a clinical psychologist at Hawaii State Hospital in 1966, was able to develop a prototype of age measures that I named the Hawaii Age Test (HAT). It consisted of a cumbersome procedure involving eight measures. After many years of testing and retesting to ensure the validity and reliability of my results, I was able to convert this procedure into a quick and simple examination.

It has been demonstrated that there are more than forty characteristics that progress reliably with aging: systolic blood pressure (the force with which the heart pumps blood), respiration rate, tremor, visual accommodation, adaptation to darkness, hearing loss, pitch discrimination, reaction time, dexterity coordination, dental and other skeletal changes, and glucose tolerance in the blood, to name a few. In formulating the AGE it was found that not all these characteristics had to be tested to achieve reliable results. Therefore, the number of tests was whittled down. Although the ability of the eye to adapt to darkness remains an extremely good indicator of aging, it was ultimately discarded because of the high cost of measurement equipment and the length of time needed to administer the test. Strength and speed tasks lacked the sensitivity to pinpoint body age to the nearest year. Blood and urine measures that involved painful, costly and often time-consuming analysis were also eliminated.

In the end, the measures that remained and were considered to be the most relevant for the AGE included five auxiliary tests— finger dexterity, glucose tolerance, cholesterol level in the blood, and peridontal and dental decay indices (which record the number of missing and decayed teeth). These are optional components to a basic, three-part examination that measures hearing level at high frequency, near vision threshold (the ability to read print up close) and systolic blood pressure. The final result is a body age that represents the middle score of all three tests. The exam is simple, portable, totally painless and can be conducted in 10 to *15* minutes.

Initial AGE investigations using National Health Survey figures turned up some interesting facts. Women, it seemed, aged more slowly than men until they reached a calendar age of *50*. Under the age of 50, the body age of women averaged as much as 13 years younger than that of men. However, at 50 calendar years the female body age caught up to the male's, exceeding it by an average of 4 years and more after the age of 60. Women seemed to grow older

Looking at the Family Album

most quickly between 40 and 50, their bodies aging 23 years on the average during one decade. Between 50 and 60 they continued to age 5 years faster than men. Dental decay and glucose tolerance tests revealed that women aged more quickly than men in those areas but had an edge over men on systolic blood pressure, high-frequency hearing and peridontal health, until they reached the age of 50.

Clear differences also emerged between blacks and whites. The two races were equal in body age until 21, but the biggest jump occurred between 21 and 30 calendar years, when the bodies of black men were 5 years older than those of their white counterparts. Between 30 and 60 the difference became even greater. Only on the dental index did whites age more rapidly than blacks. Serious tooth decay for the average black person did not begin until 40, whereas whites normally suffered serious problems by the age of 21.

These findings were highly suggestive. Why did women seem to age so much more rapidly than men between the ages of 40 and 60? Do menopause, the accumulated but delayed effects of childbirth, cosmetic deterioration, marital insecurity, raising adolescents etc., tie into this? What about the extra 5 years of physical age black men suffer in their first decade of adulthood— by inference, a particularly damaging time of life? All these questions are still begging for answers.

The response to my work was encouraging. An independent insurance company began discussions as to the usefulness of measuring body age for the purpose of offering reduced insurance rates to those with low scores. However, subsequent economic reversals made the company unwilling to reduce rates for anyone.

An engaging offer came from a prominent attorney in the United States who wanted to aid one of his clients, a pilots' union, which was attempting to change its policy of forced retirement at 60 for its members. Never having been in favor of forced retirement, I suggested to him that, in addition to a stiff physical, an annual checkup could include body age measurement. With a satisfactory physical and a body age test registering below 60, a pilot might well be allowed to continue flying. But I thought the union also should know that if the body age were *over* 60, management could retire the pilots *before* they reached the chronological age of 60. I think this only fair; I'd rather not fly with a pilot who has aged prematurely to

Growing Younger

the point where the AGE rates him at past 60. I heard nothing further from the attorney or his client.

How to Take the Adult Growth Examination

You do not have to be a psychologist or a physician to administer the Adult Growth Examination. But you may wish to consult these professionals to interpret the results of the tests. (One woman who scored poorly on the hearing test subsequently consulted her doctor who discovered that she was suffering from an ear infection. Once it had cleared up, she was tested again and her hearing had much improved.) For the AGE to be administered satisfactorily, you must be familiar with the test materials and carefully follow instructions. Some skills in psychological testing and some previous knowledge of the subject of gerontology might be helpful. Yet, after practicing under supervision, any intelligent adult will be able to monitor her or his own body age as well as that of friends and family members. The tests may be used professionally by psychologists, physicians, mental health workers, nurses, researchers and other specialists in the fields of health or life sciences. A complete manual including step-by-step instructions, score sheets and exact equipment specifications can be found at the end of this book.

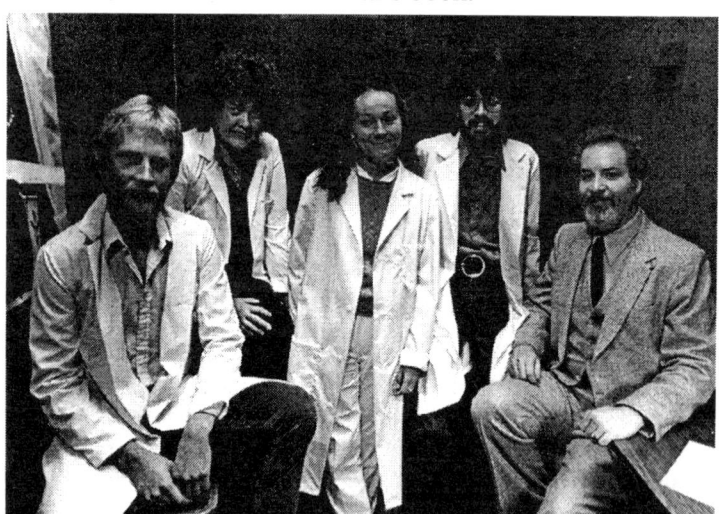

Above, AGE research team. From left: Wayne Oake, Joy Spears, Sheila Connolly, Tom Malcomson, Robert Morgan.
Photograph by Dwight Storring.

Looking at the Family Album

Your set-up for testing doesn't need to be elaborate; my own AGE lab at Wilfrid Laurier University was a small, windowless room furnished with a bookcase, a table, a lamp and two chairs, besides the actual equipment. Some of my volunteers arrived wearing sweat suits and carrying a change of clothing, expecting to be submitted to a rigorous stress experiment. That's not what AGE is all about. Most people can be tested in 10 to 15 minutes, but being relaxed is more important than observing a time limit and the results are bound to be more accurate.

In order to administer the AGE you need three pieces of equipment. These can be found in most schools and health clinics.
1. A blood pressure monitor to measure blood pressure. These battery operated machines with solid-state circuitry allow rapid, accurate measurement without a stethoscope. Or you can ask your doctor to measure your blood pressure when you have your next check-up. If you wish to acquire your own monitor, however, some models are quite inexpensive, but the preferred kind may cost $150 or more.
2. A portable audiometric monitor (Beltone, for example), to measure high-frequency hearing. This equipment may cost twice as much as the blood pressure monitor. It operates on normal AC wall current and is equipped with solid-state circuitry, stereo earphones, a microphone and a variable volume dial.
3. A portable visual near-point indicator to measure visual acuity. Use a rule that expands to 65 inches and a set of target cards that you can print yourself on a 10-point type typewriter.

Systolic blood pressure is measured first. The readings record blood pressure when the heart beats. Three readings are taken: one at the beginning of the session and again after each of the other two examinations. The second test measures hearing loss at high frequencies—6,000 cycles per second—for the better ear.

Pure tones at varying decibel intensities ranging from 0 to 110 are broadcast. through the earphones of the portable audiometer. Beginning with a frequency high enough for the tone to be heard (usually 50 db), intensity is gradually decreased until a level is reached at which you miss the tone about half of the time. Once this level is confirmed by retesting at 5 db above and 5 db below it, it is recorded.

The third test records the closest distance for uncorrected binocular vision (no glasses) at which a printed sentence can be read

Growing Younger

without blurring.

With the help of charts drawn up just for this purpose, the raw hearing and visual test scores and the average of three blood pressure readings are converted to the body age scores. Total body age is the median or middle measure of the three scores.

For example, Mrs. T takes a body age test. Using the score sheets and tables in the back of this book we can compute her body age as follows:

- Her three blood pressure readings are 118, 128 and 126; the average is 124. Her blood pressure age is 41 years.
- She needs at least 10 decibels of sound to hear a high-frequency tone on the audiometer. Her hearing age is 45 years.
- On the visual near-point indicator, the words on a target card begin to blur when the card is drawn 11.4 inches from her nose. Her near-vision age is 44 years.

Mrs. T has scored 41, 44 and 45; the middle score is 44. Her body age is 44 years. If her husband's readings on all three tests were the same, he would score a blood pressure age of 27, a hearing age of 28 and a vision age of 44. Mr. T's body age would be 28.

Occasionally, someone comes to our lab to be tested but is unable to take all three AGE'S, possibly because of equipment failure or physical disability (for example, blindness). These negative factors should not stand in the way of arriving at a body age score since a combination of at least two tests will still produce viable results.

The three-part test is reliable within 5 years above or below the body age score. No one will have a specific body age score below 19 or above 71, and most people will score a body age (BA) within 10 years of their chronological age (CA).
1. BA the same as CA: about 7% (1 out of every 14 tested).
2. BA within 10 years of CA: about 67% (2 out of every 3 tested).
3. BA within five years of CA: about 47% (1 out of every 2 tested).
4. BA more than 10 years older than CA: about 16'/2% (1 out of every 6 tested).
5. BA more than 10 years younger than CA: about 16½% (1out of every 6 tested).

Neither in theory nor in fact are body age and chronological age always synonymous in the AGE. Any valid body-aging test probably would show most people to be within 5 or 10 years of their calendar age; in only a few instances would these ages be identical. Many would show a discrepancy greater than a decade.

Looking at the Family Album

Basic Measures

What is your Blood Pressure Age?
To get your systolic (maximum) blood pressure, take the average of three readings several minutes apart. If you don't have a portable monitor, ask your doctor to give you a blood pressure reading the next time you have a physical. Take the average of three readings and compare your blood pressure with the age scores.

Age	Men	Women
21	122	112
30	125	116
40	129	123
50	134	134
60	144	141
70	148	160

How is your Hearing? I said, HOW IS YOUR HEARING?
The audiometer measures the amount of volume you need to hear a high-pitched tone of 6,000 cycles per second. A tone of 6,000 cycles is about equal to the sound from a shrill whistle. Like all high frequencies, unless such tones are exceedingly loud, they become harder to hear as we grow older. Loudness is measured in decibels.

Age	Men	Women
21	+05	+00
30	+11	+04
40	+16	+07
50	+22	+12
60	+38	+21
70	+52	+27

How is your Vision?
At age 21, you should be able to hold a newspaper to within 4 inches of your eyes (without glasses) before the print starts to blur. Also for 21-year-olds, the number of teeth missing, filled or decayed should be no more than 14.

At 30, you should be able to bring the paper up to within 5½ inches of your eyes before the blur starts. As we grow older, we become more long-sighted. We begin to see only distant objects

Growing Younger

clearly while those close up tend to appear fuzzy.

At 40, the circle of fuzziness spreads to within 9 inches of your eyes. The teeth casualty score is up to 18 in men, 20 in women. As arteries harden, blood pressure goes up to 129 in men, 123 in women. To hear the same sound you heard at 30 will take 5 more decibels.

You're 50, and the paper gets fuzzy when you bring it to within 15 inches of your eyes. A more serious loss of vision sets in around now. You need two or four times more volume to hear the same sound you could hear at 30. The sugar level in your blood is up 25% from when you were 21.

At 60, the paper blurs within 39 inches of your eyes. Dental casualty score is 24 for men, 26 for women. The chance of peridontal disease is four times as great as it was when you were 21. You likely have corns on your toes, a bit of arthritis and itchy skin. But if you hang in there for another 5 years, you'll pay reduced prices at the movies.

Auxiliary Measures

What is your Blood Glucose Level?
Your doctor can measure the amount of sugar in your bloodstream. An hour before the test, you will drink a sugar cocktail consisting of 50 grams of sugar in 250 cc (about a shotglass full) of water. This test measures how effectively your body uses up sugar, an ability that rapidly declines with age: Measured in milligrams per cubic centimetre:

Age	Men	Women
21	95	104
30	102	110
40	115	118
50	118	133
60	130	145
70	140	160
77	155	179

What is your Dental Casualty Score?
You can get this one from your dentist. Find out how many of your 32 permanent teeth are missing, filled or have a cavity. Then match your score against the average shown below.

Age	Men	Women
21	14	14
30	16	18
40	18	20
50	21	22
60	24	26
70	27	28

What is your Peridontal Index?
This is another one for your dentist to compute. Peridontal disease erodes the gums and the base of the teeth. It increases with age. A peridontal index is the dentist's way of measuring the average score of the disease's progression for all your teeth.

Age	Men	Women
21	0.6	0.5
30	0.9	0.6
40	1.3	0.8
50	1.6	1.2
60	2.2	1.6

What is your Serum Cholesterol Level?
Your doctor can test this easily by measuring the amount of cholesterol (a waxy white substance) present in your blood stream. Cholesterol in. the body increases with age and is thought to contribute to hardening of the arteries. Measured in milligrams per millilitre of blood.

Age	Men	Women
21	179	186
30	207	198
40	228	214
50	231	238
60	234	262

How Dextrous are your Fingers?
See the testing manual at the back of the book for an explanation of how to score this one.

Growing Younger

TOM MALCOMSON was a 26-year-old student researcher working on a master's degree in experimental psychology at Wilfrid Laurier University. He had been administering body age tests in our lab for more than a year.

Tom first tested on the AGE at 26—exactly the same as his chronological age. But his hearing level was equivalent to that of a 52 year old, a fact he found shocking. At first he blamed it on his 5 year membership in a noisy rock band, but he soon realized that he had been under a fair degree of stress for several months. His father had died shortly before the testing, and he had broken a long-term relationship with a woman.

When he was retested seven months later, his hearing level had dropped to age 19; indeed, his body age had dropped to 19 as well. He recalls that he was reasonably happy and content at that time.

Tom says he can usually guess the body age of the volunteers who venture into our AGE lab, but in two instances he remembers being completely wrong. The first instance was a "little old man," who despite his smiling perky face, seemed to have a very frail and old-looking body. His shoulders were stooped, his gait was slow and he took small and child-like steps.

On the form he had been asked to complete before the test, he had left the space for his birth date blank, refusing to divulge his age until later.

When Tom looked at the readings he noticed that the scores were fairly young. The man smiled when Tom told him that he had a body age of 45.

"I am 79 years old and very proud of it," he told Tom. "I fought in World War Two and always have been physically active doing things outdoors." He also had a positive attitude to life. "The world goes on," he said, "and I'm not going to let it get me down."

The second case involved an elderly woman from the United States who was attending a summer study program for senior citizens at the University. Tom recalls that she was very skinny, her hair was thinning and her complexion so pale that it looked as if it had never been exposed to the sun. She seemed to be out of breath when she arrived at the AGE lab.

"If I would have had to bet on anyone not being younger than her chronological age or at least ten years older, I would have picked her," said Tom. "I wondered how I would break the news to her, since everyone else in her group had tested out at their own age or five to ten years younger."

However, her systolic blood pressure was 19 years; her hearing was incredibly good; and she tested out at a body age of 20, but was 68 years old!

"What's more, she *told* me she lived on beer and potato chips, liked chocolate and never did much exercise. Her positive attitude must have kept her young," said Tom.

"Of course, all those in the group who had survived past their retirement age did have a healthy sense of humor. Multiple-casualty had struck again! I guess if you're doing enough things right, a few wrongs can slip by," Tom told us with a shrug.

~

The Nova Scotia Test

An AGE test was performed on a group of 107 paid volunteers from Nova Scotia. Although the subjects, 51 men and 56 women, ranged in years from 20 to 70, their average age was 40. They were representative of the average population of that province and had similar economic status and levels of education.

Before the test all the volunteers had to complete a background information sheet. They then took the basic 10-minute Adult Growth Examination. Afterwards they were asked what they thought their body age would be.

Seven percent of the volunteers showed identical body and calendar ages. Fifty percent had a body age older than that registered on their birth certificates and 43% were younger. Two-thirds of the volunteers had bodies that were within 10 years of their calendar ages on either the plus or minus side.

In the final analysis, the average body age for the 107 volunteers was the same as their average chronological age — 40 years. But the average of their estimated body ages was lower — 35 years. Ninety-three percent of the subjects underestimated the difference between the years they had lived and the age of their bodies, regardless of direction, whereas only 7% estimated their body ages correctly to the year.

Two women born 40 years before the test took place registered

Growing Younger

at body ages of 19 and 60 respectively. Both looked their body age; however, the factors that differentiated them from others like them need to be explained in greater detail.

The volunteers were divided into three groups—rapid agers, normal agers and slow agers. By comparing the idiosyncrasies of these groups, some factors generally associated with longevity soon became evident.

The body age of the rapid agers was at least a decade older than their calendar age. The eight women and two men who made up this group had a mean calendar age of 46, which was very close to their estimated body age (47 years). But their tested body age on average was actually 61 years (range 53 to 71 plus). (See Table One.)

Table I. Nova Scotia Test—Both Sexes

Analysis of Slow, Normal, and Rapid Age Rate Groups Age in Years by Birth (Chronological Age—CA), by Measurement (Body Age—BA), by Self Estimate (Estimated Age—EA)

Age rate group:	"Young" Slow Agers	Normal Agers	"Older" Rapid Agers
Number of people	9	18	10
Average CA:	53	52	46
Average BA:	38	52	61
Average EA:	47	52	47
CA range:	40-60	40-60	40-60
BA range:	19-49	35-65	53-71+
EA range:	30-60	32-60	35-55
Mean difference from CA: BA-CA:	-15	0	+15
EA-CA:	-6	0	+1
Mean difference from BA: CA-BA:	+15	0	-15
EA-BA:	+9	0	+14

Additional note on EA: using CA as a reference point, none of the "young" slow agers estimated themselves *older* than their birth age while "older" rapid agers estimated themselves *younger* than their birth age in only 20% of their group. Thus incidence of mistaken direction of aging was low in both slow and rapid age rate groups.

Table 2. Nova Scotia Test—Both Sexes

Analysis of Slow, Normal, and Rapid Age Rate Groups Selected Differentiating Factors From Questionnaire Data

Age rate group:	"Young" Slow Agers	Normal Agers	"Older" Rapid Agers
Number of people	9	18	10
% Females:	44	56	80
Median Annual Income	$ 6,000	$ 6,000	$3,881
Maximum Annual Income	$20,000	$15,000	$6,000
Lifetime Happiness	78%	67%	40%
Present Happiness	44%	44%	50%
Median Number of Cigarettes Smoked per week over Lifetime	0	0	50

The body age of the slow agers was at least a decade younger than their calendar age. Two women and seven men with an average calendar age of 53 years qualified. They had estimated, on average, that their bodies were 47 years old, the same as the rapid agers. Yet their tested mean body age was 38 years (range 19 to 49).

For purposes of comparison, the body age of the normal aging group was within 5 years of calendar age. The calendar age, body age and estimated age of members of this group averaged 52 years. This comparison is revealing. Note that 100% of the slow agers and 80% of the rapid agers already knew the direction their aging had taken, although they had underestimated it. Also, the normal aging group was quite accurate in its estimates, and virtually all the rapid agers could easily be distinguished from the normal agers, and again from the slow agers, by their appearance and behavior. The signs probably were as clear to the individuals concerned as to the observers. (See Table Two.)

To merit definitive conclusions many more Adult Growth Examinations would have to be carried out. However, the results achieved in the Nova Scotia Test proved to be consistent with more ambitious longevity studies. We now can state with some certainty that rapidly aging adults often are in a lower economic bracket than normal and slow agers; they smoke more, and many characterize

Growing Younger

their life as unhappy rather than happy. In none of the three groups did marital status, religion, health, job satisfaction and alcohol consumption influence the results.

We continue to gather information through research on the factors that influence us as we grow older or younger, faster or slower.

If you are eager to test and score your own body age, consult the *Adult Growth Examination Manual* at the end of this book.

Expected Relationship Between Birth Age and Body Age

1. Birth age the same as body age: about 7% (1 in 14) of those tested.
2. Birth age within 10 years of body age: about 67% (2 in 3) of those tested.
3. Birth age within 5 years of body age: about 47% (1 in 2) of those tested.
4. Body age more than 10 years *older* than birth age: about 16½% (1 in 6) of those tested.
5. Body age more than 10 years *younger* than birth age: about 16½% (1 in 6) of those tested.

~3~
Looking at
HYPNOSIS
The Elkind Effect

"INVESTIGATIONS attempting to reverse aging patterns and discover analogues of aging processes have not been popular with psychologists, although the potential benefit from such research is self-evident. In this age when we are called upon to be 'relevant' there are few areas of investigation which are more necessary."

More than three decades have passed since that mild reprimand was issued by psychologist Jack Botwinick, yet with some notable exceptions, it remains, unfortunately, an accurate description.

Leonard Elkind is such an exception. A skilled hypnotist and clinical psychologist, he was the first to use the Adult Growth Examination as a measure in his attempt to reverse the aging process. Working with women between the ages of 39 and 53, Elkind found that in just one hypnotic session he could implant positive thoughts about youth and vitality, thereby reducing his subjects' body age by an average of 11 years within four weeks. With this dramatic demonstration he became the first to scientifically illuminate the potential impact of hypnosis on aging.

Elkind now runs a successful private practice from his home in San Diego, using hypnosis and self-hypnosis to help people function at a higher level intellectually, emotionally and physically. Whether his clients want to improve their health, their work or leisure pursuits, he helps them see themselves as comfortable and relaxed individuals functioning at the highest level of their potential.

To meet Leonard Elkind and to hear him lecture, you might conclude that he never stops practicing hypnosis. In front of a university class of about 100 students and professionals he talks about

Growing Younger

hypnosis and aging in a deliberately soft and mellow voice. By slowly moving back and forth in front of the blackboard, he seems to mimic the swing of a pendulum. He relaxes his audience to make them more receptive to new ideas. He believes that "teachers, doctors, dentists — perhaps even parents—should all learn hypnosis techniques for the benefit of their students, patients and children."

I met Elkind in Hawaii in the '60s when I was a psychologist in private practice, in addition to doing some consulting work in the University of Hawaii's Peace Corps project. His interest in using the AGE to measure possible body changes following hypnotic suggestion grew out of his extensive knowledge of things related to the body — athletics, massage, psycho-therapeutic techniques, bioenergetics, the martial arts and yoga — all based on the concept of energy flow through the body. His premise is that physical and emotional trauma leads to a blocking of that energy flow, inhibiting structures on an emotional and physical level. If the energy could be freed, the body's natural flow would be restored. Hypnosis is a technique that speaks to the part of the mind that regulates the body. Twinning it with the AGE seems to be the natural route to follow, so that the way the mind might influence body age could be measured.

It is not yet possible to either fully define or adequately explain hypnosis. The word entered the language about 100 years ago to describe a natural state of mind that exists in everyone from birth. As we grow up, most of us lose the ability to slip into the relaxed, imaginative subconscious state of our mind. Hypnosis is akin to daydreaming. You can be entranced by a movie you see or a book you read and you can believe that what is happening on the screen or on the page is real enough to make you cry or roar with laughter. Hypnosis is a state of physical and mental relaxation during which your mind is open. In a sense it is like a child's game, in which by using your imagination you have access to your subconscious.

Hypnosis draws on the side of the brain that controls the involuntary or autonomic nervous system and the intuitive, creative part of your mind. On that side of the brain our breathing, heartbeat, body temperature, and the size of our pupils are regulated.

Elkind read his first book on hypnosis about 30 years ago, when he was in his first year of high school, and calls self-hypnosis the most powerful tool capable of intervening in the aging process. He believes that all hypnosis is self-hypnosis, but what a therapist does is help put his subject into a better hypnotic state.

Looking at Hypnosis

According to Elkind, hypnosis is merely limited by our own imagination and ingenuity and by the skills of the hypnotist. His research with the AGE demonstrates that by tapping into the subconscious mind incredible changes in the body and the conscious mind can take place. People may see their bodies as naturally healthy; under hypnosis he tells them that they will feel that their bodies are healthier, and that they will experience a sense of energy and a tingling sensation when they breathe.

Most of us incorporate negative hypnotic suggestions throughout our lives. We wind up thinking that we can't do or are afraid to do certain things, or even that we're going to die of a heart attack. Most of Elkind's work is geared toward silencing these negative voices within us. If we, so to speak, get out of our own way, our bodies will return to their naturally healthy and vital states.

Aging is a source of anxiety for most of us. Elkind calls the four little words, "How old are you?" one of the most emotionally loaded questions. The popular concept of growing old can be so depressing to some people that a significant number of them would prefer to die prematurely rather than face the prospect of aging.

Elkind points to the newsstands for reinforcement of this fear. A full-page magazine advertisement, accompanied by a photograph of a smiling woman and an obviously doting man, sports the parenthetic comment, "He forgets I am 50!"

> "Isn't it wonderful to read about getting to look more youthful, and know it can happen to you? Isn't it comforting to be able to realize that you are about to see the last of age-making facial lines for many a long year, if ever again, and that skin dryness may become a total stranger to you from now on? These blessings can be bestowed upon any woman over 25, for little more than just the asking!
>
> After age 25, in the female, the cells of the skin usually begin to shrink in size due to reduced ability to obtain water and retain it. Skin then dries and "falls in". These areas are the lines that are so worrisome because lines can become wrinkles that give the "over 35" look a grasp on appearance that is difficult to break.
>
> This is not a dream about the mythical "Fountain of Youth". Scientific and medical journals have acclaimed this startling discovery, called CEF (Cellular Expansion Factor), as the first real break-through to renewed beauty for women of all ages."

Growing Younger

Such advertising is a major thrust in the anti-aging campaign, preying on and reinforcing the fear of growing older. Another more recent example by Clairol, Inc. shows a somewhat more subtle and perhaps even more insidious approach.

> "After all the time you spend trying to look younger than you are, your gray-haired husband is unintentionally telling people your age. Causing all that vanity to be in vain. Well, Clairol can once again help you look younger, and it isn't with a new lipstick, or a new conditioner, or a new eyeliner. It's with a new hair coloring. For men. (Obviously, if your husband looks younger, you'll look younger.)"

Perhaps more to the point than the question, "How old are you?" is the question Elkind asks: "How old are you, really?" It is generally accepted that people age physically at different rates. Human aging is a complex process involving a great deal of intense emotion; relatively little is clear in the way of systematic explanation. Some people doubt that aging and death are natural.

The idea of reversing the aging process is not a new one. There are a great many physicians, psychologists and sociologists who theorize that aging is not entirely the result of physiological factors; that death itself may be the result of mental factors, such as attitude. A good deal of research has been done on the consequences of fear, "voodoo" curses, and other psychogenic causes' of death as a result of the expectation of dying. Self-fulfilling prophecies create an expectation of decreased ability and vitality with increasing years.

According to Elkind, "the psychosomatic aspects of health have been discussed by many people in widely differing contexts. Socrates, in perhaps one of the first allusions to the body-mind relationship, pointed out in 500 B.C. that there is no illness of the body apart from the mind' and that it is obvious that the body could not be cured without the mind."

In building up to his experiment with hypnosis and the AGE, Elkind found that the gap between the conscious and the unconscious mind could be narrowed in many ways. Ultimately, he based his work with the AGE on four fundamentals:
1. Physical aging should not be taken for granted.
2. The idea of reversing the aging process is not widely accepted but neither is it new.
3. Hypnosis has been used in past experiments to affect some

of the same measures that are used in the AGE.
4. The body and the mind are inexorably linked.

Following these fundamentals, Elkind points out that disciples of yoga believe that the body as well as the mind are naturally suggestible; that there is a vital energy stored in the body, which can be tapped to overcome the deterioration process we expect to encounter with old age.

Paul de Sainte Colombe has used "graphotherapy" as a therapeutic technique that can alter a person's handwriting to bring about character and personality changes. He believes that handwriting is a physical manifestation of subconscious attitudes. Others use meditative techniques to come in contact with the life pulse by focusing on the rhythmic -beating of the heart or meditating on color to produce physical effects.

Ramanand, a Yogi has shown that it is possible to control basic functions within the body, something generally accepted to be beyond conscious control. Results of a study in New Delhi confirmed the yogi's ability to slow his heart rate at will, to decrease his consumption of oxygen to one-quarter of the minimum supposedly required to maintain life, and to cause perspiration to appear at one point of the body only (the forehead).

Scientists have been able to train animals and people to control their autonomic nervous systems; for example, their heart rate, blood pressure, constriction of muscles in the tail, the ears or the stomach, the rate of contractions of the intestines, and the rate of formation of urine. Psychologist Neal Miller also has trained patients with rapid and irregular heartbeat to slow down their heart rate; those with high blood pressure were able to reduce their readings through thought control. He worked with conditioning techniques, using a tone as a reward for changing the blood pressure in the right direction. He also had some success in training epileptics to suppress the abnormal electrical activity of the brain, which is characteristic of their condition.

Similar physiological control methods and change through hypnosis have been demonstrated by others, but many of the findings are contradictory and inconclusive. One of the first and most remarkable experiments was carried out by James Esdaile, a British surgeon working in a prison hospital in India from 1843-1847. He used hypnosis as the only anesthetic to perform more than 3,000 operations, of which more than 300 involved major surgery. Prior to this experiment half of Esdaile's patients died, a statistic considered normal in those days. After he began using hypnotic anesthesia, however, his mortality rate dropped to only 5%. When Esdaile returned to England, he was persecuted and called blasphemous by fellow doctors for his attempts to control pain. He was subsequently tried by the British Medical Association and deprived of his license to practice.

Of particular interest in modern times are the effects of experiments following the hypnotic state itself. Children with hearing loss have benefited by direct suggestion under hypnosis. Hypnosis also has been shown to improve visual acuity. One case involved a myopic medical intern who under hypnosis regressed to an earlier age, when he was able to wear glasses appropriate to that particular chronological age. Subsequent regression to an age prior to the onset of his need to wear glasses allowed him to dispense with them entirely. Unfortunately, no attempt was made to carry his achievement over into the waking state, despite the intern's own repeated and unsuccessful attempts to attain the same results.

In Dr. Elkind's doctoral thesis for the California School of Professional Psychology, he set out to see whether hypnosis could effect a lasting measurable change in the body. On the assumption that the unconscious mind holds knowledge capable of bringing about a decrease in body age as reflected by the AGE, Elkind used hypnosis to implant suggestions of youthfulness in the subconscious minds of his voluntary subjects.

Nineteen women ranging in age from 39 to 56 took part in the tests. Initially they were all subjected to the AGE and it was found that their body ages ranged from 23 to 66. The group was then divided. Nine women underwent hypnosis one week after their first AGE test. At the beginning of the session, they were told the following:

> We are here today to explore two aspects of hypnosis. The first is the induction of hypnosis and for this we will be using a standard hypnotic procedure that I will be reading to you. Trance *induction* is one thing, and trance utilization is another, just as surgical preparation and anesthesia are one thing, and the surgery is another. Hypnotic *induction* is a preliminary to *utilization* of the hypnotic state, which belongs to another category of behaviour, and is the sec-

ond area of interest for us. I will be saying things that are general enough to meet the needs of *all* of you, and things specific enough to meet the particular needs of one of you.

First, you will experience a wide range of hypnotic states as an *induction,* then a *still more* personal experience of how they can be *utilized* to achieve satisfaction of your own needs.

Just as when you have an interesting conversation or watch a good movie and time passes without you realizing it, the time today may prove to be as interesting and absorbing. At times, you may notice that your willingness to go deeply fluctuates: sometimes a little, sometimes a lot. If this happens, when *you* feel very ready, take two deep breaths, and go deeply relaxed.

People have many different kinds of experiences in hypnosis and many people find it hard to tell after a little while, whether they are in hypnosis or awake. Don't try to do anything, or not to do anything, just let yourself go. Just let it happen.

This "pre-talk" set the stage for post-hypnotic suggestion and answers to common questions:
1. Why is it so simple?
2. Why hasn't it happened yet?

It also served to broaden the subject's concept of hypnosis and to create a doubt that she was actually aware of her own state of mind.

After this brief question-and-answer session Elkind inserted the following suggestions:

Remain deeply relaxed and pay close attention to what I am going to tell you next. Now, when you came into this room you brought into it *both of your minds,* that is your conscious and your unconscious mind. Now, I really don't care if you listen to me with your conscious mind, because it doesn't understand this anyway, so I just want to talk to your unconscious mind because it's here and close enough to hear me, so you can let your conscious mind listen to the noises here in the room. Or you can think about any thoughts that come into your conscious mind, systematic thoughts, random thoughts, because *all I want to do is talk with your unconscious mind and it will listen to me* because it is within hearing distance even if *your conscious mind does get bored. Just be comfortable while I am talking to your unconscious mind since I don't care what your conscious mind does.*

Your conscious mind is your thinking mind. Your unconscious mind does its own thinking, but not always in agreement with your conscious mind. The unconscious mind is a positive force which will arrange what is best for you if you stop interfering with it. For example, to begin to pay attention to walking causes you to stumble, while to leave walking to the unconscious means easy movement.

Listen carefully to my words. All you have to do is hear them. Your unconscious mind will receive and understand their meaning and will give that message of renewed *vitality* to your body.

The body is a self-repairing organism. Wounds heal by themselves. When you get a cut, you let air get to it and your body knows how to repair the damage. Change for the better is a natural development. Everyone knows that it is natural to feel *vital* and *healthy.* Through hypnosis your body can become *younger,* not like a child but like a healthy, vigorous adult. You may wonder how this can be so.

Hypnosis speaks directly to the unconscious part of your mind. The part that takes care of healing cuts, that makes you perspire, has you digest your food, has you sleep and dream and many other things that are beneficial to you.

How does your body remember? The unconscious has its own memories, such as never forgetting how to ride a bicycle. I'm tapping your unconscious mind on the shoulder just like your memory needs to be reminded. I am using hypnosis to help your unconscious mind *utilize* its knowledge of healing, to remember how you feel when *you* feel young.

Allow your body to heal itself. You have a wonderful

capacity for rejuvenation within you. Let yourself feel *younger,* more *vital.* Feel the *vigor* and *health* that is yours. Your body is built for hard use. All you have to do is *relax* and allow your body to take care of itself. Others of your age will seem somehow much older than you are.

You will be more attuned to the world around you. Things will be *clearer, easier to understand.* When you are tired you *rest;* when you are worried you *relax;* you know how to feel *renewed.* Just as you can get older over a long time, you can be rejuvenated in a short time. Just as a new idea may strike like a bolt of lightning and change a person's life forever, these thoughts and your increased youthfulness will last far into the future. Expect it to be enduring.

The induction was then completed. A brief discussion of the experience revealed that the women had found it pleasant and were interested in taking part in hypnosis again.

All nineteen subjects were retested on the AGE in the fourth week after the start of the experiment and three weeks after the hypnosis session. Half the women in the control group showed a decrease in body age and the other half registered an increase. All women who had undergone hypnosis showed a decrease in body age, from 3 to 18 years. Also, hypnotic susceptibility (as indicated by their responses to the standardized Harvard Group Scale of hypnotic susceptibility), did not influence the degree of body age change.

Spontaneous comments by the women who had undergone hypnosis after their second AGE test indicated that many of them felt they had entered a different state of hypnosis when suggestions of youthfulness were introduced. Some said they had been interested, but not entirely involved, until then. Additionally, some reported they had occasionally experienced a self-hypnotic or daydream-like state in which they heard suggestions for youthfulness, saw themselves as younger, thinner and more attractive, or had "a cathartic release of pent-up energy." One woman, who thought she hadn't been hypnotized, was quite concerned that she wouldn't enjoy the benefits of the suggestions for youthfulness because she could not remember having heard them.

Growing Younger

Table 1. Scores for Subjects Under the Control Condition

Subject	Ca[a]	BA-1[b]	BA-2[c]	BA Difference
1	39	26	22	-4
2	41	38	40	+2
3	44	45	46	+1
4	44	33	30	-3
5	45	42	41	-1
6	46	50	53	+3
7	46	59	55	-4
8	47	50	51	+1
9	50	53	52	-1
10	56	48	52	+4
Median	45.5	46.5	48.5	0

[a]Chronological Age
[b]First Body Age Test
[c]Second Body Age Test

Table 2. Scores for Subjects Under the Experimental Condition

Subject	Ca[a]	BA-1[b]	BA-2[c]	BA Difference	HS[d]
11	39	45	28	-17	9
12	40	37	20	-17	8
13	41	23	20	-3	5
14	41	37	30	-7	8
15	44	40	22	-18	5[e]
16	44	59	49	-10	11[e]
17	47	30	19	-11	2
18	49	66	50	-16	5
19	53	50	44	-6	9
Median	44	40	28	-11	

[a]Chronological Age
[b]First Body Age Test
[c]Second Body Age Test
[d]Hypnotic Susceptibility (self-rating on the Harvard Group Scale of Hypnotic Susceptibility, Form A)
[e]Prior experience with hypnosis

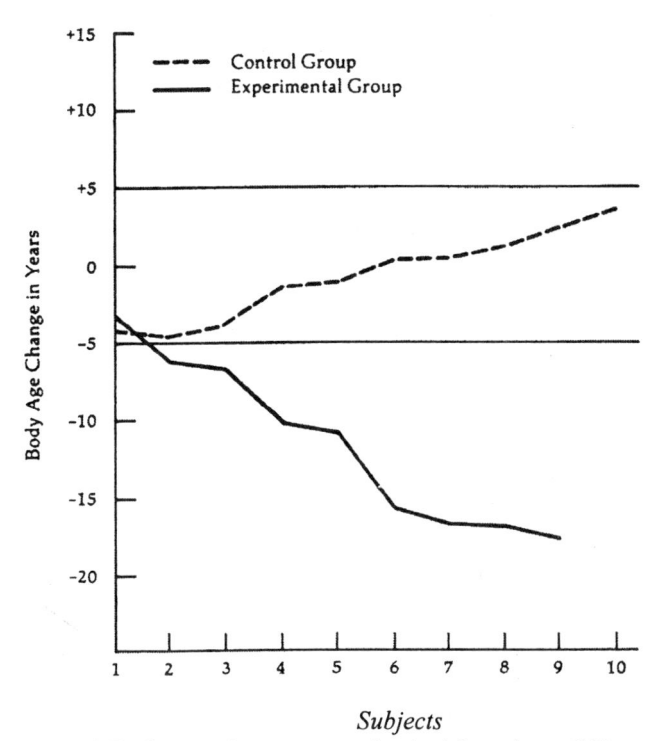

Figure 1. Body age change scores (ranked from least difference to between first and second testing). The -5 to +5 area represents the standard error of measurement of the AGE.

The experimental group, however, showed eight of the nine subjects with body age change scores beyond the -5 standard error of measurement. As may be seen from the data in Table 2, the subject with the body age change score of -3 years (Subject 1) was a 41-year-old woman who scored a BA of 23 on the initial testing and a BA of 20 on the second testing. As the lower limit of the AGE is a BA of 19, insufficient room remained for her to show significant change.

The study did not determine why these women's body age scores had dropped, nor did it set out to do such an investigation. However, there is some justification for assuming that the women who had volunteered represented the sort of group that would seek remedial treatment of the kind offered in the experiment. Whether everyone would benefit is a matter for further study. Tables 1 and 2 on page 37 show the results of the tests in more detail.

Figure 1 represents the ranked body age change scores for subjects in both the experimental and control group. As may be seen from the diagram, all of the body age change scores of the control group fell between the -5 and +5 boundaries of the standard error of measurements of the AGE. Therefore, none of these individual changes were considered significant.

Elkind was surprised at how well the experiment had worked after just one session with hypnotic suggestion. He had anticipated having to coax hidden data, but there it was, all laid out right in front of him. Since there was no follow-up, Elkind had no scientific data to indicate whether the effects were lasting, but he did get some anecdotal evidence that the hypnosis had produced long-term results.

The woman whose age had dropped the most on the test was "relatively nondescript, a brown-and-gray person. In the study she was just going along, intellectually there, but you wouldn't describe her as full of life. And she was somebody who was not particularly impressed with the work at all." She was 44 years old at the time of the study and initially tested at a body age' of 40. After hypnosis she had a body age of 22—a drop of 18 years. Elkind saw her again several years later. "It was amazing," he said. "As though she were a different person. She was dressed differently, looked younger, her eyes were brighter and she seemed to have a lot of respect for herself. She was much more dynamic, full of life, talking and enjoying herself."

In his present work, Elkind continues to use the lessons he learned with the AGE. He tries to build positive concepts about health, youth and vigor regardless of whether clients come to him for help to quit smoking, to lose weight or to enhance their lives in some other way. He believes that people normally function at between 5 and 15% of their true capacity, and therefore he attempts to help them tap the other 85 to 95%.

I used Elkind's techniques to measure body age change in my own lab. Here is the case of a 59-year-old woman who, within the space of a couple of months, managed to drop her body age from 61 to 40.

~

Looking at Hypnosis

MARG MESTON is a quiet-spoken university secretary who plays a mean hand of bridge during her lunch hour. She is a mother and grandmother who loves to read, hates to do housework, but characterizes herself as a relaxed person, "maybe too relaxed." But she suffers a touch of arthritis.

I wanted a volunteer to undergo the AGE testing in connection with a hypnosis demonstration of the Elkind Effect to implant suggestions of youthfulness and vigor into a subject. A Canadian network television show *(Live It Up)* wanted to film the procedure to discover how it worked and Marg volunteered. Although she was interested in hypnosis from a medical point of view and could see that it could have benefits in relieving tension in childbirth and, perhaps, dentistry, she didn't really know what it was all about. She had read about hypnosis in the newspaper and had seen it done on the stage.

Marg's first body age test pinpointed her at 61—well within the normal range for her chronological age. Then she and Alan Edmonds, the television journalist, and his crew went to the office of Dr. Victor Rausch, a local dentist who uses hypnosis extensively in his work. Several years earlier, Rausch himself had undergone gall bladder surgery while in a self-induced hypnotic trance. No anesthetics or drugs had been used and he had walked from the operating theater to his hospital room under his own steam. The anesthetist who had accompanied him called the procedure "unbelievable, unless you were there."

He now was to hypnotize Marg and implant suggestions of youthfulness, health and vigor in her mind, carefully following the procedure laid down by Dr. Leonard Elkind. "I sat in a comfortable chair," Marg recalled, "the television lights were on—they were warm and comforting—and the camera was rolling. It was dead quiet. Dr. Rausch, sitting at my shoulder, started talking to me. I closed my eyes and he lifted my hand off the arm of the chair. It fell back down. He kept lifting it until finally, it stayed up in the air. Then he began to tell me that I was going to feel younger and more alert and not to let things bother me. There was a lot of repetition of his words, which lasted for about 10 or 15 minutes. Then he told me I would open my eyes at the count of five. I did."

Growing Younger

Dr. Rausch later reported that Marg had been in a state of deep relaxation. By using rhythms in the tone of his voice and by touching her shoulder, wrist and forehead, he tried to condition her mind to be more susceptible to suggestion. His signal that Marg was not paying attention to her body came when her hand no longer fell back onto the arm of the chair. He then repeated over and over again that she had control of her body, that it would regenerate itself, become younger, energize easily and that she would achieve a balance that was both physical and mental. He created images, using the color blue to suggest a mist that was drifting all around her. He asked her to let herself be covered by it, to breathe it in so that it would flow through her body as if it were a vital energy. He told her that when she opened her eyes she would feel relaxed and refreshed, and be alert and awake without tension. He then clapped Marg's hand back onto the chair and she opened her eyes.

Marg's arthritis continued to act up for two weeks. Then it went into remission. Three weeks after the hypnosis she was retested on the AGE. Her score was now 50—a drop of 11 years. She was tested again six weeks later and had a body age of 40. Asked about this remarkable change, Marg admitted she was puzzled.

"But I find it very interesting," she said. "Maybe it was the hypnosis. I feel exactly the same, and don't think I've changed in any way. I really don't know what to think...."

~

Hypnosis may prove to be the most powerful tool we have to mitigate the aging process. Currently, much of our lives is governed by preconceived notions about what we are capable of and how we should behave and function as we grow older. We believe that as the years pass, our bodies are supposed to break down; our memory, eyesight, and hearing are expected to fade and our sex drive to wane. But people who learn to relax and are taught not to unconditionally accept these myths about aging have the choice to reject such "prescribed" deterioration.

~4~
Looking in
THE MIRROR
Self Programming

ASK YOURSELF these very personal questions: What will I die from and when? What did my parents and grandparents die from and at what age? Do I fear the same will happen to me?

The answers you provide will form the basis of a powerful and basic psychological aging concept—the Self-Fulfilling Prophecy. Some of it will be rooted in your childhood, through suggestions implanted by your parents or your school experience. But it may also stem from your peer group or even from yourself. The same concept has been applied to research and the classroom and our expectations can influence the outcome just as much as teachers' expectations of student performance can influence the test results of student learning. The existential concept that we create our own world is applied here with serious consequences. Deep hypnosis is only one variety of the continuing programming we all undergo as part of our contemporary life, and if we concede that the mind is rooted in the body, the pre-programmed thought will naturally affect the way our bodies work.

Here is one example of how such pre-programming works with children. Some of us who do public consultation in clinical or counseling psychology occasionally run across insomniacs who, when they were young children, recited the mandatory bed-time prayer that went, ...and if I die before I wake... To illustrate how this may affect adults, let me quote from one of Gene Schoenfeld's ("Dr. Hip Pocrates") write-in cases. Dr. Schoenfeld's column appeared in the *Berkeley Barb* in the late 1960s and early 1970s.

> *Dear Dr. Schoenfeld:* I'm 22 years old and have been going with the most far-out girl for the past 5 years. We've been smoking pot for about 3 years but only in moderation. My problem started last January when my sister (who's straight) showed me an article in the paper really putting down pot. Just for laughs I read it, a move that I've regretted ever since. It said that pot smoking creates impotency in some males. For 5 years we've been getting it on 2 to 5 times a week, but the very first time we tried after I read that article, it was "no show." I realize that the only thing that is wrong with me is that I've lost my confidence, but how am I supposed to get it back? If that girl leaves me they're going to have to put me away. I don't have the bread to see a shrink and we've been rejected by the local family counseling service because we're not married yet.
>
> *Answer:* Many "free clinics" have psychological counseling services or you could call the department of mental health or your local mental health department for a referral. But since you seem to have reacted to a newspaper article perhaps you'll respond also to this one. Wesley Hall, president of the American Medical Association, has said that marijuana "makes a man of 35 sexually like a man of 70." Later he admitted there was no evidence for this statement but if his words reduced marijuana use he has accomplished his purpose. In other words, Dr. Hall has "gotcha."

Lawrence Casler, a gerontologist who has applied the principle of self-fulfilling prophecy to aging, has also attempted to manipulate it. He states that "many physicians, psychologists and sociologists have long believed that the diminished vitality so often accompanying the aging process is not entirely the result of physiological factors. Indeed, death itself may stem from nonorganic causes. Concentration camp prisoners who died because, reportedly, they had lost the will to live, and deaths in other societies occasioned by 'voodoo' curses and the consequent expectation of dying, are only a few examples that might be cited to suggest that death may have a psychosomatic component."

Casler also observed that there are forms of behavior expected of individuals at specific age levels. For the elderly these include a notion of gradually decreasing vitality terminating in death. Cultural norms and social pressures combine to induce the individual to behave in a fairly stereotyped manner and to ingrain the virtually inescapable notion that he or she should die no later than whatever age limit is culturally prescribed. These pressures begin early in life, when youngsters are taught to regard their grandparents as feeble and to respect their frailties. But the aged individual himself who sees people around him—his war buddies, brothers and sisters, neighbors and friends—becoming ill and dying, focuses those expectations most strongly on himself, to the point where no alternatives may seem possible.

Casler set out to investigate whether, among older people, changes in these attitudes could modify or reverse their preconceived notions about aging. He visited the Jewish Home and Hospital for the Aged in New York City and recruited 30 volunteers who agreed to let him help them enjoy life more. To do that he divided his subjects into two groups, matched for age, sex, physical and mental health and length of residence in the home. The average age was 83 years. (More than half were European Jews who had come to the United States in the late 1930s and early 1940s.) Casler proceeded to visit each of the 15 volunteers in the experimental group at least five times over a period of five weeks. The other 15 were to be a control group.

Although the subjects had looked forward to his visits, he was not able to apply his planned technique to all of them. In the few cases where he was able to put his original plan into practice, he would ask the individuals to sit or lie back comfortably; next he would use a standard method to help them relax more deeply, and then proceed with the following suggestions:

> A person is as young as he feels. You may have many happy, healthy years ahead of you — years full of opportunities for pursuing your interests and hobbies and developing new ones, making new friends and enjoying life free of financial and other responsibilities. You will find it easy to relax, to enjoy yourself and to remain healthy and happy for many years to come.

Casler elaborated on these phrases and repeated them over and over again. Afterwards some of the subjects would remark that they felt refreshed and relaxed, and expressed a desire to implement the suggestions in their everyday lives.

The experimental subjects who had refused to cooperate with Casler wanted to tell him about their families, neighbors or their own lives instead of sitting or lying quietly while he did the talking. Yet, whenever possible, he tried to interject his message, which although differing from person to person and from week to week, essentially remained the same: advanced age need not be accompanied by debilitation, helplessness or demoralization. Some accepted his message readily; others were resistant and some emerged unconvinced.

One year after the sessions had ended, Casler compared the illness and hospitalization rates of the experimental group, whom he had visited and attempted to help, with the control group, who had not received his positive suggestions about health and wellbeing. He found that 19 of the volunteers had been sent to hospital for periods ranging from a few days to several months— 10 from the control group and 9 from the experimental group. The control group had been confined to hospital for a collective 1,346 days, while the experimental subjects had only spent 974 days there. The average for the controls was 134.6 days; 108.2 for the experimentals. Three from the control group and two of the experimental subjects were permanently transferred to a hospital. Excluding them, the averages dropped to 47.2 days and 24.7 days for control and experimental subjects respectively.

The differences become even more dramatic when the death rates are compared. Six of the 15 controls (40%) died within a year of the experiment. Only one member of the experimentals died (7%).

Here are Casler's conclusions:

Should these trends continue, the implications are rather exciting to contemplate. It may well be that by means of suggestions similar to those I have described, it will be possible to improve the health, happiness and manageability of residents of old age homes. Viewed more broadly, these trends suggest that we reconsider our usual notions of aging and the determinants of death. A person who expects to become helpless or to die at the age of 80, 85, or 90, is likely to have his expectation confirmed. The process is closely akin to what has been termed the "self-fulfilling prophecy." By counteracting these expectations, at least to some extent, the types of suggestions I have been giving may be institutionalized, self-fulfilling prophecies of their own. Needless to say, this study will raise more questions than it will answer. It is quite possible, for example, that the suggestions were irrelevant; all that was necessary was the weekly chat with an attentive, relatively younger person. No one advocates a long life, *per se,* if the advancing years impose upon the individual a totally dependent, vegetative existence. But long life, accompanied by vigor, joy, perhaps even a little passion — this is consummation devoutly to be wished.

In 1981, Casler released a 15-year follow-up study on the old-age home volunteers. He found that those who had received positive verbal suggestions concerning health and longevity survived more than four times as many subsequent years as the residents who did not receive the suggestions (8 *vs.* 2 years). Those who did receive them also spent four times as many days without hospitalization over their remaining years.

Earlier, Casler had taken his work one giant step further. In 1970 he served notice that he had begun a long-term study that would take a lifetime to complete. He had recruited 100 volunteer college students to study the effects of hypnotic suggestion on longevity. One-half of the volunteers were given suggestions unrelated to longevity, while the other half were receiving forceful statements emphasizing that people did not have to die at a certain age and could live to be at least 120 with all their mental and physical faculties intact. When the study was initiated the volunteers were all about 20 years old. Obviously, final results will not be available for about 100 years, but Casler fully expects to present the results himself at that time. I therefore wrote to him asking if he had undergone hypnosis himself. No, he had not, he replied. He felt that strong suggestion and belief were sufficient; the fact that he was a poor hypnotic subject would not matter.

Growing Younger

Samuel J. Warner, in his book *Self-Realization and Self-Defeat,* does a nice job of illustrating the power of the self-fulfilling prophecy. He claims, for example, that a child who receives attention from important adults only when he is hurt may soon learn to become "accident-prone"— to win by losing. This kind of basic learning is acknowledged by most psychological frameworks, be they Skinnerian, Freudian or eclectic.

Early learning may be the basis for many programmed suggestions, life scripts and self-fulfilling prophecies. While the child is developing a self-identity, he is profoundly influenced by the people close to him, the people he likes to imitate. We have long known that parental example is more potent than parental advice. Most parents are models for the adult their child will become. Of course, some children may choose to remodel as adults, but most do not.

Let us now look at another significant facet of longevity. Data show longer life for those born to younger parents. Since the mother is the more important person for this effect, it would seem that very early infancy may well be the time for the child's aging processes to be imprinted. In fact, infants may model their own adulthood on the first adult they synchronize with and perceive. If this is so, changing aging expectations, possibly by hypnotizing a young adult, may reverse any disadvantage in longevity accruing to those born of older parents. This, of course, is still speculation awaiting testing.

Do we, in fact, have an expectation of when we are to die? There is evidence for this, of both a situational and an internalized origin. Let us first look at the situational.

A graduate student at a psychology professional school was also a priest. He described a retirement home complex paid for by his brotherhood as "luxurious." As time went on, the apartments filled up and retired brothers had their names put on a waiting list. The wait, of course, was for someone in an apartment to die so that a new occupant might move in. As the waiting list grew longer, the situational pressure grew stronger. Several residents of the luxury apartments remarked to my informant that beyond a few years' residence, they felt guilty about keeping the space for themselves; beyond five years they definitely felt death to be an honorable expectation. Most met this expectation.

Many old folks' and retirement homes encourage the same ex-

Looking in the Mirror

pectation. The average person dies about seven years after retirement. The mortality rate is highest during the first few months spent in an institution for the aged. I am convinced that if young adults in their late teens and early twenties were subjected to similar conditions (no visitors but family; you are treated as being at the end of life) the mortality could approach that now recorded for senescents.

Biofeedback has demonstrated that we can control our heart, temperature and other body processes. Expectation based on suggestion may be the trigger. Is suggestion the same as hypnosis? Opinions on the definition of hypnosis are far from unanimous. In sex research and practice, an increasingly prevalent treatment is to enlarge breast size through hypnosis. Women are regressed to the age at which their breasts were developing to re-experience them growing; then, when projected ahead in time, they visualize the larger breasts they desire. It was reported that the technique generally yielded a two-inch gain or more, but the success was enhanced when the subjects monitored their own progress. In effect, the degree of success depends upon how much responsibility people will take for their own development.

In line with this finding, one school of hypnosis feels that since all hypnosis is effective auto-suggestion, we decide for ourselves which suggestions we ought to internalize. Leslie LeCron and David Cheek, the leading exponents of this approach, therefore advocate conscious awareness of this process through deliberate training in the skills of auto-hypnosis or self-programming. Dr. Cheek, a gynecologist and obstetrician, has contributed much to our understanding of hypnosis for several decades. His research in the early 1960s demonstrated that people under stress (including anesthetized patients) are in a hypnotic state triggered by their situation, and are extremely prone to incorporate suggestions and comments made by people talking in the vicinity. By the same token, doctors and nurses, by careless or pessimistic conversations during an operation, could harm or even kill the patient. To use this finding more productively, deliberately optimistic comments were made during operations to reduce morbidity by as much as 95%. Dr. Cheek went on to investigate the effects of stress, particularly illness, on conscious patients. He found hypnosis (direct suggestion) through self-hypnosis to be effective in reducing symptoms (from hemorrhage to respiration) and emotional resistance to getting well. Focusing on obstetrics, he developed a technique for reducing birth mortality and increasing maternal satisfaction by regressing pregnant mothers to relive their own delivery, as perceived from the safe emotional vantage point of an observing adult. This time the mother re-experienced the consequences of good and bad delivery practices. In this context, mothers recommended optimal birth conditions such as soft lights, music, etc. Dr. Cheek's work prefaced Frederick LeBoyer's "birth without violence" techniques, first espoused in 1975. Whereas LeBoyer was motivated by empathy and humanism, Cheek was additionally motivated by the mothers' own recalled experiences and their preferences for birthing environment. With this technique it was also possible to determine pre-programmed self-fulfilling prophecies about childbirth and change them for the better, wherever they had been destructive.

Cheek therefore demonstrated that hypnosis, if defined as extreme sensitivity to suggestion, is a much more pervasive phenomenon than is generally realized. Furthermore, suggestions made at critical times may become internalized and self-perpetuating. Finally, the expectations may be re-programmed by a competent professional hypnotist or, with proper training, by the persons themselves.

I was delighted to be able to recruit David Cheek throughout the early 1970s to teach his techniques to graduate students in psychology. Veterans of his classes learned to use hypnosis for a variety of purposes—from speed reading to greater self-awareness. Many explored their past by verifying parental conversations, occasionally to the embarrassment of parents. One woman remembered (through auto-hypnosis) a discussion between her parents when they were on their way to the hospital where she was subsequently delivered. "Father complained loudly that they were just not ready to have another child," she recalled. Thirty years later, a surprised and embarrassed mother verified the story to her daughter. Such seemingly magical memory has a reasonably scientific basis, because the infant's cortical structure is intact before birth. Several months before delivery, the infant can vocalize, kick and demonstrate basic learning. While it is doubtful that the child can comprehend what it hears, the cortical system can store the sounds, subject to recall at a later date via hypnosis or by other means. Infant and even pre-natal programming takes place, usually without adults being aware they are doing it. (Psychiatrist Tom Veiny's recent book, *The Secret Life of Your Unborn Child,* is probably the best summary of this point of view.)

One psychology student in Dr. Cheek's class began to recall her early years during quiet times at home. Once she chose to see what she looked like at the age of 3 by retrieving a memory of her 3-year-old self looking in the mirror. "I recognized that it could be difficult to look very unselfconsciously in a mirror again," she said. "An older version of myself might well be looking back." She also used the Cheek method to train her "photographic memory" which was particularly useful for exams. Such use is really a function of transpersonal or human potentials psychology. But how does all this apply to aging?

Undoubtedly we all have expectations about it that can be recognized and reprogrammed via hypnosis and autohypnosis. See if *you* can visualize how long you expect to live. Try to see an exact number. Meditation and hypnosis might help if you cannot come up with a number. You might try to enhance this visualization by lying down, holding your head very still, and looking into a pair of goggles that have white paper taped over the visor. Most people can visualize clearly under these conditions. Once you know how *you* are programmed you can choose to develop a new expectation. You may also monitor your success with the AGE measurement procedure.

The infant's self-concept programming, as it affects longevity and aging, may be termed a form of psychological heredity. If heart attacks run in your family, aside from any inherited congenital malformation, there likely will be an inherited expectation to contend with and to disengage from. Long term studies of blood pressure in children, for example, generally show a high correlation of child and mother by the age of 6 months. Adopted children show the same correlation although they take somewhat longer.

Ask yourself what same-sex ancestors in your family have traditionally died from. At times, identification with an adult is so great that anxiety grows the closer you get to the age this adult was when he or she died. This is known as the "anniversary neurosis." Elvis

Growing Younger

Presley died at an age identical to the death age of his mother, with whom he had strongly identified. In clinical jargon, anniversary neuroses may be found in most of us at one time or another. What are yours?

We see much in contemporary life that reflects mortality programming. Phillip Kunz, a Brigham Young University sociologist, took a random sample of 747 obituaries published in Salt Lake City during the one year checking the dates of death against the decedents' birthdays. Forty-six percent of all deaths occurred in the three months following the birthday while only 8% came in the three months preceding it. More than three of every four deaths occurred in the half-year following the birthday. Why are people six times as likely to die in the three-month period following a birthday rather than before it? Kunz feels that although most people deliberately or unconsciously choose to reach the cultural milestone of another birthday, they get so depressed and unmotivated to go on, once that goal has been reached, that they die. In terms of the self-fulfilling prophecy, this may be more evidence that with or without depression, internal programming will carry us to a specific birthday but not much farther.

The power of the brain to destroy or protect the body is becoming more apparent to modern science. Nicholas Cummings, the founding president of psychology's first professional school, was also chief psychologist of a health services organization in northern California. As part of his job, he hoped to evaluate the impact of psychology on his organization. From the financial and human resources point of view, he determined that it could ill afford to forego psychological services. A patient receiving two to eight interviews with a psychologist usually averaged a 75% reduction in medical utilization over a 5-year period; one session alone could reduce medical utilization by 60% over the same period. The implications for any national health insurance plan are obvious. It has long been recognized by a majority of physicians that many, perhaps most, outpatients are more in need of a good listener than of medical pharmacology or surgery. Moving from general practice, we now see psychologists and psychiatrists becoming involved in the prevention of death from mass killers such as cancer and heart disease.

Is cancer psychosomatic? If we believe in multiple causation,

then surely expectation is one possibility worth tracking. Researchers in this area have isolated personality factors predisposing cancer, heart disease and other important causes of death. The key factors predisposing one to cancer include:
—harboring resentment and blocking anger
—self pity
—poor self-image
—inability to maintain long-term relationships
—the final trigger is usually depression caused by a great loss or setback.

One hypnotic approach, taken when cancer has actually begun, uses the visual imagery of bodily defenses attacking the cancer; heart disease also is now being treated this way. Effective prevention will, of course, affect longevity as well as hospital utilization. Aging itself demands more attention from an approach that encourages people to take charge of their lives and bodies in a positive way.

In the area of human potentials, we again see expectations determining results. Gertrude Schmeidler's classic work on extrasensory perception in 1952 and 1954 demonstrated this effectively. People who did not believe in ESP did significantly worse than chance could account for. Her approach remains one of the most reproducible lab experiments in both psychic research and the demonstration of the self-fulfilling prophecy. Here is how you can demonstrate this:

Find a volunteer who adamantly asserts that ESP is nonsense but is willing to be tested anyway. He must be rigid and forceful in his belief. Have him sit with his back to you while you flip a coin twenty times. He calls heads or tails each time. By chance alone, you would expect him to be correct about half the time. In fact what frequently happens is that all or nearly all his calls will be incorrect, a result far beyond the normally accepted limits of coincidence. This negative ability is called "psi missing" but a better term would be "psi negative" since ESP is being used in a self-defeating way to maintain a sad self-fulfilling prophecy. (I have seen the experiment used at parties and it rarely seems to fail.)

A conversation with one of the AGE lab volunteers shows how

expectations can creep into our everyday lives. Some people may be willing to passively accept and abide by them; others may make a conscious effort to fight against them.

~

MARLENE is a lively and attractive 35-year-old "superwoman," an energetic individual raising thirteen children (aged 5 months to 17 years), nine of whom are biologically her own. She is completing a bachelor of arts degree in psychology and is thinking of entering medical school sometime in the future. In the spring months, when she has some spare time, she runs a custom drapery business in her home.

The living room of her large downtown home on a tree-lined street is an oasis of calm in a bustling household. A cake-icing ritual is underway in the kitchen and her children wander in and out of the house with their friends while Marlene, dressed in jeans, her hair held back in a bun, feeds the 5-month-old baby a bottle. (Note: The baby is her daughter's.)

She has taken my aging course and was tested six times on the AGE. "Before my first test," she says jokingly, "I entertained the idea of buying shares in Memory Gardens in case I was right off the scale."

A friend who was tested with her the first time said she was an ardent women's liberationist who thought a woman's body should not be polluted and misshapen by having babies. Marlene, too, considers herself a feminist, but with a totally different attitude. She says that she "was going to be damned" if she proved on the test that having kids "wiped you out of the female race."

Marlene tested at a body age of 20. Since then she AGE tested five times at 19, the lowest score possible.

Asked to comment on these results, she had both pragmatic and philosophical answers. "It may have to do in part with my genes. My father was an alcoholic who abused his body all his life; he is still alive at 70. My mother is working full time at 65 and runs part of a farm. My grandfather lived through two world wars to be 99.

"I've always taken a fair amount of pride in keeping physically

Looking in the Mirror

fit. With a large family everyone expects you to weigh 300 pounds and be terminally ill. But you don't sit on your butt when you're taking care of a family this size," she says.

According to some standard longevity predictors, Marlene says she should be dead "in five minutes." She was born to an older mother and her parents divorced when she was 14. Her family moved around a lot while she was growing up. She had her first child at age 17. "Everybody expected me to fall apart."

"The day you are born, there is no guarantee that everything is going to go perfectly well every day of your life. I expect the kids to get into fights at school. I get onto teachers because I don't agree with some of the things they do. It's all part of living. There's no shot you can get that will give you immunity from life."

How does Marlene handle stress?

"I don't consider a lot of things stressful that other people do, such as physical work, for example." Marlene intends to enjoy her life.

When one of her teenage daughters became pregnant, Marlene decided she would help her daughter raise the child in her own home, "to turn a negative situation into a positive learning experience." She also fosters two children who were formerly in institutions and another who comes from an abusive and alcoholic family. "I tend to get very excited about issues, especially the treatment of children and school systems," she says with conviction.

"I feel very much alive. I don't think of myself as 35, but as 15 years smarter than I was at 20."

~

Self-Programming Exercises
— Using the techniques suggested in this chapter, speculate on when your life will end and how. If you do not wish to accept these expectations, decide on a set of new ones and try to imprint them in your mind (through meditation, professional hypnosis, or just plain determination). See if this procedure affects your body age.
— Can you use autohypnosis to affect your body age? To determine some of your early programming? To change internalized expectations?
— What self-fulfilling prophecies can you discover in yourself and

Growing Younger

in others? Where did they originate? How can you change those that are undesirable?

—How could you apply the information you now have to develop a school (or pre-school) program for children so that they may develop only healthy pro-life, self-fulfilling prophecies and expectations?

—Should children be hypnotized or programmed to resist being hypnotized and programmed?

—If you were to tell people just before they are AGE tested that they looked very young, would it affect their body age scores? How about the converse?

—What is your image of an ideal self: body age, weight, height, health and ability? How can you measure your progress to reach that ideal?

~5~
Looking at
NUTRITION
Eating and Aging

DIETARY APPROACHES to better health and longer life are so effectively promoted and accepted on such a massive scale that genuinely good nutrition becomes lost in the midst of fads. Today, pseudo-nutrition is big business. Drugs, herbs, vitamins, minerals and abstinences are so intensely promoted that people with a healthy sense of skepticism cannot help but back away from them. My own preference is to base best guesses on scientifically backed research. The aging process, as we have seen, can be effectively verified through animal research or by using human tissues in test tubes.

All aging may be viewed from a cellular perspective. Yet, there are alternative ways of looking at the process. Environment, genetic programming, and what you eat and drink can affect cell longevity. Sensory and nerve cells tie all the cells together.

Let's shift the spotlight from the outside to the inside; from expectation to circulation, and from the internalization of the self-fulfilling prophecy to the internalization of the self-fulfilling pharmacy.

The effect of diet on health, vitality, longevity and aging has long been the arena for the "physician's prescription book." In 1975 we had Dr. Cantor's "Longevity Diet," in which the eminent proctologist from Flushing, New York shared his wisdom with us by giving us an anti-aging safflower oil diet. Long before that, in 1883, Dr. R.V. Pierce in his *People's Common Sense Medical Advisor* provided anti-aging counsel for that era's generation by stating that:

The diet... should be largely composed of those articles rich in the non-nitrogenized or carbonaceous elements. Fat meats, rich, sweet cream, good butter and other similar articles of diet, should largely be eaten. By furnishing the elements for the production of animal heat, they counteract the predisposition to take cold....

Dr. Pierce was President of the World's Dispensary Medical Association and founder of the then acclaimed Invalid's Hotel in Buffalo, New York. Of course, his advice would be rejected by most of today's doctors and nutritionists. Yet what his work has in common with books published right up to the present is the lack of grounding in what may be called well-designed research. The "prescription" comes from those tried and true medical standard bearers: force of authority, credentials and personal experience. Departing from this tradition, the information presented in this chapter will be based primarily on controlled studies.

Most research on aging interventions deals with diet, drugs, vitamins and minerals. After months of sifting through the most scientifically grounded material, one can conclude that in fact, we know much more about what accelerates aging than what slows it down. There are few surprises as to what these clearly destructive substances are, since they are all promoted continually by their manufacturers to appeal to our desire for pleasure. Of course, I refer to cigarettes, cigars, alcohol, coffee, refined sugar and the illegal drugs of the opium family. Caffeine and smoking can raise blood sugar levels as much as refined sugar. According to the American Heart Association, heart disease accounts for half of all diseases in the United States; smoking one pack a day will quintuple (increase by five times) the risk of suffering a stroke. But, quite likely, you know all this.

And yet, what conference (including medical or collegial) is held nowadays without the vittles being offered including coffee, doughnuts, cigarettes and alcohol? Most people, bombarded by these demonstrably noxious (and even addictive) substances, will conform to social pressure and partake in this culturally sanctioned form of population control. A campaign run by the American Heart Association offered a red, delicious-looking heart-shaped lollipop to Heart Fund contributors. Of course, many adults will show restraint by feeding this life shortening substance to their children! If you are as fully conditioned as I am to enjoy sweets, the picture need not be totally grim. Rather than practicing monastic abstinence, many people now are moving to the use of sweets that are less demonstrably harmful. I recommend the many Pritikin program cookbooks or *The Good Goodies: Recipes for Natural Snacks 'n' Sweets* by Dworkin and Dworkin. Blended bananas or a few of the non-carcinogenic sugar substitutes such as sorbitol are reasonable sweeteners.

The McCay Method

In 1927, Cornell nutritionist Clive M. McCay began his classic dietary experiments to control the life span of rats by balancing the composition and quantity of their diets. Before examining the effects of these diets, which varied in specific proportions of protein, carbohydrates etc., Dr. McCay mapped out a mini-study to isolate the effect of bulk on longevity. He randomly assigned a litter of rats to either an experimental or a control group, once they had been weaned. The control group received a normal diet of rat crunchies and water; the experimental group was fed only the essential proteins, minerals, and vitamins. Control rats were allowed to eat "ad lib" (whenever they chose) an unlimited food supply, including sugar and lard as well as the essentials. McCay felt that underfeeding the experimental group might retard their growth rate and, consequently, extend their longevity.

The control group averaged a normal life span with the longest-lived rat lasting 964 days (about 96 human years). Those. in the experimental group generally lived about twice as long as the controls, their longest-lived member lasting to 1,320 days, the equivalent of about 132 human years. When fed ad lib at 1,000 days, they experienced a spurt in growth; females were able to have litters even at that advanced age. The underfed rats were furry and vigorous long after the controls had died, and when they finally expired they did so as a result of such things as brittle bones—causes that most rats do not live long enough to experience.

The actual diet used for the underfed animals was high in proteins and vitamins, specifically: casein 40%, cooked starch 22%, lard 10%, sucrose 10%, salt 6%, cottonseed oil 5%, cellulose 2%, 15 units vitamin A, and ¹A gram yeast (D). McCay later endorsed brewer's yeast, whole wheat flour, wheat germ, liver, eggs, milk, calcium and vitamin B1 as beneficial for human consumption. Unlike the many "prescription" endorsements made during the past century, his were based on decades of thorough research.

Although he did go on to other experiments, the underfeeding treatment was the most explosive one to assist the budding science of gerontology. McCay had clearly demonstrated that there was no unchangeable species-specific average or maximum lifespan. The rate of growth affected aging and longevity; smaller size and body weight correlated with greater longevity. Underfed rats older than 1,000 days were "centenarians," with most of the characteristics of young rats still present, including intelligence, high activity rate and glossy coats. They were, however, slightly smaller than normal rats and some, on McCay's diet, developed osteoporosis (loss of calcium in the bones) and calcification in the aorta or kidneys. Further, growth had to continue at least at a minimal rate or death would occur. Aging continued with underfed rats; it was merely slowed by a factor of two or three. The technique proved valid on mice as well as on rats, and it was not necessary to block sexual maturation to accomplish extended longevity. In human terms, we have here a treatment that, if applicable, promises to produce centenarians with the appearance and vigor of teenagers. Unfortunately for those of us old enough to read this, the McCay Effect is much reduced if it is not begun in childhood.

All over the world, other laboratories based experiments on McCay's work. In one later replication the oldest surviving rat lived to 1,465 days, which is about three times the normal average life span of McCay's control rats.

A decade after McCay's initial work, another group of researchers looked at the effect of fasting with the intention of prolonging the lives of rats. At weaning, they were randomly assigned to one of three groups: no fasting, fasting one of every two days, fasting one of every three days. Males that fasted lived 20% longer and fasting females an average of 15% longer. The group that fasted every other day lived slightly longer than the one that fasted every third day. None of the "fasters" experienced drastic growth retardation, as had McCay's rats, and the development of tumors was retarded in direct proportion to the amount of fasting. The longest-lived rat died at 1,073 days. It now was known that fasting in itself could extend the lifespan without negative effects and that the McCay Effect could be attributed to much more than going without food.

Scientists further explored the incidence and growth of tumors for underfed rats. Again, using the McCay technique of caloric restriction, they found that at the end of two years, the McCay rats were five times as likely to be tumor free, but they also were smaller than the controls.

Caloric restriction has been tested on dogs with the same results. The canines showed a reduction in chronic diseases as well as greater length of life. The application of these findings to all mammals, including man, now had greater credibility.

We now know that reduced caloric intake in rats need not lead to stunted growth or blocked sexual maturation. In human terms this means that underfeeding need not create a generation of asexual Peter Pans, forever 13, who take decades to grow up. Most of us would pass up being 13 for decades, but would consider remaining 23 a more attractive possibility.

The earlier in life that weight is reduced, the greater the impact on longevity. But this effect will only occur if weight reduction is instituted before maturity.

There are critical ages at which post-weaning caloric restriction operates at maximum potency. Translating rat days into equivalent human years, the best food distribution is:

0—2 years   —Nursing
2—7 years   —Ad lib feeding, high quantity of food, especially protein
7—32 years   —Reduced caloric intake, reduced protein
32—50 years —Further reduced caloric intake, further reduced protein
50+ years   —Maintain weight, reduce nothing

We now can see that the time that underfeeding should take place is at least as important as the underfeeding itself. Feeding should not be reduced before about 7 years of age and not after 50; "the less you eat the longer you live" (given basic diet essentials) only seems to hold true for the period of life between 7 and 50. Protein intake is best if high in early life and reduced in later life. Junk carbohydrates (sugar, pop, etc.) shorten the life span in all phases of life but especially in the period between 7 and 32 years, the age group that high-carbohydrate products are mainly sold to.

Of course, I have taken animal data and extrapolated it to humans. I realize this is a risky generalization and that more decisive data still would need to be gathered on our own species. However, at present the above study constitutes our best guess as to the effects of diet on longevity.

The Czechoslovakian physiology team of Stuchlikova, Juncova-Horakova and Deyl traced the world-wide interest in the McCay Effect by demonstrating its influence on hamsters, mice and rats. The team generated specific life-span percentage advantages (over normal feeding) for three different diets: Diet 1 consisted of half rations throughout life; Diet 2 of normal ad lib feeding when young (under one year) but half rations when old; Diet 3 of half rations when young (under one year) but normal ad lib when old. Based on work with 25 male Wistar rats, 100 golden hamsters, and 100 mice, they concluded that Diet 3 was the most potent in extending the life span, although the rats were overweight (pleasure from regaining forbidden food?), followed by Diet 2 and then Diet 1. The specific percentage of life span advantage over rodents fed normally throughout life was:

Diet #	Hamsters	Mice	Rats	
1	9%	27%	32%	Half rations throughout
2	30%	29%	43%	Ad lib young, restrict old
3	50%	38%	61%	Restricted young, ad lib old

As there was no scientifically credible treatment for actually slowing aging processes until the 1930s, it is not surprising that gerontologists seized upon the McCay Effect with even greater interest than before. Even though it took them another three decades to sufficiently recognize McCay's work, today's aging specialists can point to his approach as the promise of their science.

What will happen to his concept when applied to humans? In 1972, Duke University's School of Medicine popularized the use of what the press called "Miracle Medical Cocktails," composed of essential nutrients including glucose, salts, vitamins and amino acids. This 2,400-calorie elemental diet was served to patients suffering from complaints that ranged from gastric problems to those allergenic in nature. The low-bulk preprocessed liquid diet lightened the burden on the kidneys, liver, stomach and intestine. Asthma, hives and arthritis, as well as dangerously-high cholesterol levels, responded well to it. (The absence of caffeine, nicotine, refined sugar and alcohol undoubtedly also had an effect.)

Following extensive publicity, the diet was marketed (at about $10 per day) under the trade names "Jejeunel" (Johnson & Johnson) or "Vivonex" (Eton Laboratories) and is still available today through non-prescription channels. Vivonex comes in six different flavors (orange, vanilla, chocolate, grape, strawberry, and beef broth). If the calories were to be substantially diminished through the reduction of carbohydrates (presently 9.8% in Vivonex) while the vitamin and mineral levels were to be substantially increased (especially C, E, B5, zinc), we would have a near-prototype for the kind of diet most likely to demonstrate the McCay Effect in humans.

Vitamins and Aging

This is an area of nutrition littered with rhetoric, speculation, mystification and over-generalization that has led to a cultural blindness, especially in medical and scientific circles. True, most of the more important contributions to nutritional science rest on scientific studies with animals other than *Homo sapiens*. Perhaps the research with Adult Growth Examination and similar measurement techniques will bridge this generalization gap.

Some good classic references for promoting the strengths of these nutritional contributions include a series of books, such as *Nutrition and Vitamin Therapy* by Dr. Michael Lesser, Grove Press, *The Pritikin Program for Diet & Exercise* by Nathan Pritikin, Grosset & Dunlap, and *Supernutrition* by Dr. Richard Passwater, Dial Press. Unlike the "prescription" approach exemplified by Dr. Pierce in 1883, the authors of these books, in some cases biochemists and nutritionists, take strong positions based at least in part on solid research.

What are their conclusions? *Prevention Magazine.* summarizing the approach, recommended well-balanced meals, adequate protein, calcium, selenium, vitamins A, B complex, C, D, E, and K; and activity, sex, work and creativity at all adult ages. There is much evidence for the dietary importance of megavitamin doses of vitamins E and C, BS (pantothenic acid), brewer's yeast, nucleic acids (RNAIDNA), selenium and BHT (butylated hydroxytoluene). For example, one study with mice demonstrated a 20% increase in longevity with a 300 mg daily dosage of vitamin BS in their diets. Using injections of nucleic acids, the life span of Snell-Bagg dwarf mice (normally 3 to 5 months) was extended by more than 200%. Exercise, vitamin C, B5, niacinamide (B3), procaine hydrochloride, brewer's yeast and wheat germ in combination also have shown positive results.

Biochemist Dick Passwater traced increased incidence of heart attacks and premature aging to a lack of dietary roughage/fibre, vitamins C, E, B5, B6, minerals, selenium, zinc, magnesium, coupled with insufficient activity, increased smoking, obesity and stress. He believes that refined sugar, coffee, chocolate, cigarettes and alcohol can be responsible for developing anemia, hypoglycemia, iron and vitamin deficiency, premature aging and early death.

Pantothenic acid (B5) is mentioned in nearly all the vitamin research in connection with aging. Its discoverer, Dr. Roger Williams, found it when investigating the longevity effects of "Royal Jelly" on bees. His own studies with C-57 mice demonstrated a 19% increase in life span from a daily dosage of 0.3 mg B5 alone. On the basis of several years of research, he concluded that:

> On a purely statistical basis I would be willing to wager that if a large number of weaned babies were given 25 milligrams of extra pantothenate daily during their lifetime, their life expectations would be increased by at least 10 years. A similar bet might be made by an agronomist who, based upon his knowledge of the soil in a particular area, might wager that the corn crop on a given acreage would be increased by 10% if additional phosphate were used as fertilizer.

Williams goes on to recommend vitamins E and C since they too can affect the aging process.

The distinguished American chemist Linus Pauling popularized the concept of megadoses of vitamin C as a protector of health. Although controversy over this rages on, C does have a role as a retardant of the processes of aging; vitamin E, however, is even more potent in this regard. Where C may aid in longevity by reducing the incidence of atherosclerosis, E seems to act directly on the cell by inhibiting the accumulation of noxious granules.

Although ginseng is another controversial well-merchandised compound, it may nevertheless offer some measurable impact on the rate of aging. High quality dried aqueous extract of the herb increases cell density and hinders cell degeneration. Ginseng is not a vitamin, but the stores reputed to sell pure and high-quality vitamins are the ones where ginseng also should be purchased. Stay away from mail order ginseng; it can be made of almost anything.

Other Oral Jolts

The effects of nucleic acids continue to dominate research. These are the RNA/DNA protein chains that genetically program each of our cells. Ten 750-day-old rats (analogous perhaps to 75-year-old humans) were fed the same diets. However, half were also given weekly injections of DNA/RNA. After 12 weeks, differences in appearance, weight and alertness became obvious. The five uninjected rats died before they were 900 days of age, whereas of the five injected rats, four died at ages of 1,600 to 1,900 days, the fifth and last dying at 2,250 days! Here we have a treatment that, if replicated, could more than double the life span. Dr. Max Odens, a London physician, speculated that the cell action of the injected nucleic acids had worked primarily to prevent cancer. In studies with senile male humans to whom high-dosage RNA supplements had been given, he found that their memory had improved. An advantage over the McCay Effect seems to become apparent: aged adults seem to benefit without prior childhood application.

New York physician Dr. Benjamin Frank recommends, as rich natural sources of nucleic acids, daily doses of fish (especially sardines), fresh vegetables such as celery or onions, one multiple vitamin capsule, two glasses of skimmed milk, four glasses of water, a glass of vegetable or fruit juice, and a snack of a few ounces of unsalted nuts. He also suggests a serving of peas or lima beans once a week, and beets three times a week. He bans refined sugar, carbohydrates and saturated fats. Here, of course, is another "prescription" diet; but at least it is based on some systematic research. Dr. Frank claims that some obvious changes, such as fading age spots, do occur after several months on this diet.

Following inspection of three long-lived cultures (see chapter 7), Dr. Alexander Leaf, a Harvard University professor, suggests that beyond an intake of an ample supply of minerals and essential amino and fatty acids, aging seems to proceed at a slower rate when certain toxic substances are avoided. These include pesticides on fruits and vegetables, heavy metals such as the mercury found in some seafoods, bacterial contaminants in improperly refrigerated meats and salad dressings, and excessive quantities of salt. The average adult in our culture needs about .25 grams of salt daily, or about 3/46 teaspoonful. He overdoses on table salt by taking 40 times that amount (10 grams a day; usual range 4 to 24 grams a day). Even without using the salt shaker at every meal, the amounts contained in foods and those added while cooking are more than sufficient. Excess intake will result in high blood pressure and subsequent heart problems. Consequently, we should include reduced sodium intake in our optimal anti-aging diet.

Anti-oxidants, which slow the burnout rate of our cells, have been identified as anti-aging agents by the pioneering work of Denham Harman. Harman, the "father" of the free radical theory of aging, tested his theory through the successful use of antioxidants to protect cells from radiation, cancer, unsaturated fats, and general mortality. His rodent subjects generally experienced a 7 to 29% increase in lifespan. The anti-oxidants of his choice were the preservative chemicals MEA and BHT. MEA is 2-mercaptoethylamine hydrochloride; BHT's full name is 2, 6-di-tert-butyl-4-methyiphenol. Unlike the McCay Effect, MEA and BHT (or vitamin E) do not directly inhibit aging but rather protect the organism from age-accelerating mechanisms. Many ecology and health food proponents are unhappy about the use of these chemicals, but they do seem to have some benefits. In mice, antioxidants were effective only when the environment or the nutrition was suboptimal, a condition normal for our culture, and they seemed to function in a remedial fashion.

Some Russian scientists have developed an optimum recommended diet restraining growth, which includes anti-oxidants, complexons, megavitamin complexes, trace elements and anti-sclerotic agents. Their economy still suffers a manpower shortage, and therefore extending the productive vigorous life of their workers is to the advantage of all.

One of the more controversial drug preparations is procaine, an anti-depressant used in youth treatments by Anna Aslan in Romania. Despite the fact that American studies were better controlled, they could not replicate her beneficial results. However, the debate goes on, since subsequent articles pointed out that the preparation used in the United States differed from the European one.

Metabolism-slowing drugs like Digoxin also have shown promise and there is some evidence that estrogen, in spite of the fact that it causes some other complications, may delay by at least 10 years several aging processes, including postmenopausal osteoporosis (low bone calcium).

Protein utilization, necessary for optimal growth and age resistance, has been found to vary as much as 400% from one part of the day to the next. Based on research done with human subjects, the best protein conversion cycle may well be to eat the largest meal at breakfast time and the smallest for supper at the end of the day. Again, it looks as though those who would like to age more slowly must move directly against the mores of our culture.

Some Sample Gerontologists' Diets

A good gerontologist will tell you that a special diet should always be preceded by a good medical checkup including a lab analysis of blood, urine, and hair samples (the latter can be used to determine insufficiencies in vital minerals). You should determine before launching into them whether there is any medical reason, such as an

Growing Younger

allergy, to abstain from certain additives and food supplements. Dick Passwater proposes following a series of self-evaluation steps to determine an individual's optimal dosage of key vitamins and nutrients. Here are some of the optimal daily doses he suggests:

Vitamin A —35,000 IU (more than twice this may be toxic)
Vitamin B1 —100 mg
Vitamin B2 —100 mg
Vitamin B3 —250 mg to 3 grams
Vitamin B5 —100 mg
Vitamin B6 —100 mg
Vitamin B12—100 mcg
Vitamin C —4 grams
Vitamin E —800 IU
Vitamin D —1000 IU (2 to 4 times this amount may be toxic)

Passwater bases this "supernutrition" on health indices, primarily those that prevent illness. A good anti-aging regimen might differ from his in several respects; vitamins B5 (pantothenic acid) and E, for example, might need to be no higher for immediate health and wellbeing, but might well require larger doses to significantly affect longevity.

My own present dosage, in addition to daily basic vitamins and minerals (much like Passwater recommends), includes:

Vitamin B5 Calcium Pantothenate—4 grams (4,000 mg) time release.
Vitamin E—800 IU (half d'alpha only and half mixed tocopherals).
Vitamin C—6 grams time release (two with each meal).
Additional minerals (especially 30 mg Zinc), bone meal, lecithin, fibre, roughage, and vitamins plus natural diet rich in liquids, nucleic acids *(fish,* etc.) and devoid of caffeine, sucrose, tobacco, alcohol, and excessive fat or salt. (A good general diet is Pritikin's although I would add the vitamin and mineral supplements he foregoes.)

Looking at Nutrition

Your own best diet may well be different from this one. My children (the youngest is 11), apart from having a well balanced non-toxic diet, take a daily children's vitamin pill (non-sugar), C, E, and B5 (at a lower level than my own daily dosage). All of us eat foods that are as low as possible in fats and refined sugars. This can stimulate a good deal of kitchen creativity, especially during the hot, thirsty summer months. Instead of craving cola or ice cream, my daughters rely on freezies and other cool quenchers. Here are a few samples of easy-to-make refreshments relying on natural sweeteners.

Banana Milk
3/4 cup skim milk
1 banana
1 tsp. malt powder
1 tsp. vanilla
Blend and serve.

Freezies
Take equal amounts of white grape juice and a frozen fruit such as strawberries or blueberries. Blend and serve.

Fruit Milkshake
2 cups milk
1 cup strawberries
1 or 2 bananas
1 cup frozen blueberries
Blend and serve.

Protectively and positively, a well balanced diet and a few diet supplements can retard aging. But that in itself is not the whole story. Alcohol and coffee have now been identified as age accelerators and mortality hasteners. Blood sugar levels increase sharply with the intake of caffeine and nicotine. Dick Passwater blames the fact that 30 nations have better life expectancies than ours on our conditioned malnutrition. One of every three of our children suffer from iron-deficiency anemia. The basis for this finding is a Public Health Service study of 12,000 people in ten American states. It also

Growing Younger

revealed that one of every five adults has gross vitamin deficiencies. Passwater predicts that our median lifespan will *decrease* in the next decades (it has been constant in recent years), because of programmed inactivity, smoking, malnutrition, and air and water pollution. He points out that in 1900, one in seven deaths was due to heart disease. Today it is one in two. For those aged 25 to 44, the death rate from heart attack rose 14% between 1950 and 1970. Passwater's culprits include refined sugar, chocolate, coffee, cigarettes, alcohol, as well as reduced intake of vitamins E, C, B6, selenium, magnesium, zinc and roughage. He also abhors our incredible overdoses of table salt and toxic food additives, of which there are over 1,000 routinely used today. The annual intake increases every year. (In 1966 the intake averaged 3 pounds per American; in 1971, 4 pounds; in 1974, 5 pounds. And in 1998, 8 pounds.)

Hard drugs also remain a problem. In 1960, the estimated number of babies born to addicted mothers in New York City was 1 in 164; in 1972 it was 1 in 40—four times as prevalent.

Think of a typical Saturday you spend with your kids: you may take them to a smoke-filled circus, feed them cotton candy, ice cream cones, candy bars and salted popcorn. You yourself may have some coffee. And then it's home in the car, an hour through traffic. What a way to grow up fast!

As I reread what I've written here, I sound preachy and moralistic. That clearly is not my intent; I respect the right of individual choice, even to suicide. I think, though, that it's important that you know that you as an individual are doing the choosing. If someone had deliberately planned a high turnover rate for the average adult, it could not have been done better!

What of the future? We have heard of a successful research effort in the USSR to isolate what Russian chemical physicists call "Gero-protectors." Through the use of 2-ethyl-6-methyl-3-hydroxypyridine hydrochloride, an anti-oxidant that has been used as protection against excess radiation, the mean and maximum life spans of mice have been increased, cutting one strain's mortality by 20%.

On our own continent, we continue to make modest progress from year to year. There has been a search for a "Death Hormone" occurring naturally in our systems, and for some oral antidote to it.

Looking at Nutrition

Directions are also being taken to link lead solder and aluminum intake from defective food packaging to premature aging and health problems.

Anti-aging Ideas on Diets

Evaluate dietary changes for yourself and friends over a period of a month. This can include what you *slop* ingesting (e.g., salt, coffee, alcohol) as well as what you start to eat. See which food supplements are of value to you.

An addiction test: Can you (or your children) give up candy made from refined sugar without going through withdrawal symptoms?

Does the thought of giving up coffee or salt put you through cold turkey?

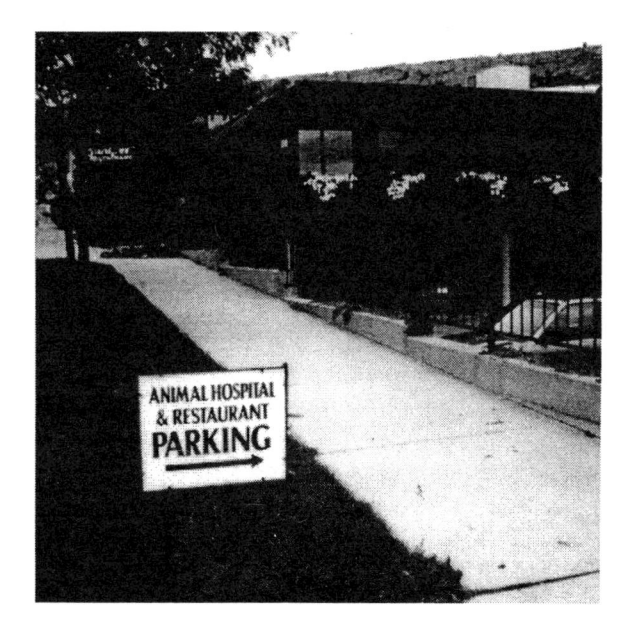

Growing Younger

~6~
Looking at
THE THERMOMETER
Metabolic Aging

IT IS NOT A NEW theory to relate metabolism to longevity. It has been suggested that animals use up the same amount of energy per unit weight independent of species life span; the more energy is used up, the more heat is produced, and therefore the shorter the life. Animals that show slow growth conserve more of their energy and live longer.

If we were to lower our body temperature, thereby slowing the metabolism, could we also slow aging? Would this be possible or healthy for humans?

Bernard Strehler, director of the Biological Laboratory at the University of Southern California's Rossmoor-Cortese Institute for the Study of Retirement and Aging, suggests that reducing body temperature by one or two degrees could add 20 years to normal life expectancy. He cites reports of fish that lived longer in cold lakes and of desert mice having low body temperatures that lived four times as long as laboratory mice. With every reduction of 15 degrees Fahrenheit in body temperature, the amount of oxygen consumption is cut in half. Dogs have been maintained at a body temperature of 92 degrees F with no apparent harm; normal humans fluctuate by one or two degrees in a regular daily cycle while those that average well below 98.6 degrees F do so without difficulty. Strehler would reset the body's thermostat in the hypothalamus for a cooler, and subsequently longer, existence. One researcher even entertained the fantasy of humans sleeping on special waterbeds to chill them at night. But it was up to Barnett Rosenberg, professor of biophysics at Michigan State University, to elucidate the full impact of lowering body temperature in humans. Using sophisticated mathematical calculations, he demonstrated that a drop to 88 degrees F, which he still considers safe, would lead to an average lifespan of 198 years; at 91 degrees F, people would average 140 years; at 95 degrees F they would live to 100 years on average. A drop of 7 Fahrenheit degrees in core body temperature could double our current average lifespan, even if such a drop were made in adult years. Rosenberg's mathematics show that if the three leading causes of death—heart attacks, cancer and vascular lesions—were prevented or cured, we could live an average of 98.8 years. However, lowering the human thermostat by even 4 degrees F would have a *greater* effect on longevity. Only past work with the McCay Effect, caloric restrictions or experiments with nucleic acids offer interventions that promise to be as potent. It may take a decade or two, just as it did with Clive McCay's work, before our culture will realize the full potential of Rosenberg's approach.

Is a slower metabolism the newly discovered fountain of youth, at last? On the contrary. In my opinion, it may be that we now have an opportunity to regain a level of functioning that was our biological potential all along, a level that has been artificially lowered by stress and the poisons in our environment. In fact absolute core body temperature, as well as being a measure of both aging rate and metabolism, can also be viewed as a sign of our reactions to the environment.

First, let us look at some contemporary alternatives to lowering body temperature. How can a mammal such as man turn down the heat? Hypothermic drugs are designed to reset our internal thermostat at a lower level rather than deactivating it altogether. But before we can look at these drugs, we need to stress that self-experimentation is *not* recommended. Particularly in dealing with prescription drugs, you must *not proceed without medical assurance* that the intake of a particular substance is safe for you. Even if the drug is legal, safe, attainable, and you have your doctor's consent, you must not attempt to reduce your core body temperature more than one or two degrees at a time and never more than a final total of 10 degrees Fahrenheit.

Enzymes (the body compounds that control chemical activity) are powerfully affected by temperature change. Although some sci-

Looking at the Thermometer

entists do speculate that people with lower body temperatures from birth may live longer, artificial change could upset the body's chemistry, particularly if it were done too rapidly. By lowering the body temperature of warm-blooded (homeothermic) mammals below 30 degrees C (86 degrees F) the risk of cardiac fibrillation (heart murmurs) is high. So there does seem to be a limit as to how far this process can safely go under present conditions. Therefore, if you wish to reduce your own body core temperature, you must make sure that:
1. The way you do it is medically safe for you.
2. You reduce the temperature very gradually (no more than one degree a day) and *you must* stop immediately if you experience any kind of discomfort.
3. Never try to adapt to a temperature lower than 88 degrees Fahrenheit.

Drug research on extending life through reduced body temperature is often very circumspect and protective about exactly which compounds are effective. Let us begin, however, with a class of drugs typically sold without prescription that many of us may have taken at times. The most commonly sold "antipyretics" (fire reducers) are Aspirin tablets. As their temperature-reducing capacities make them reasonable antidotes for high fever, they have been prescribed for years. Unfortunately, Aspirin can cause bleeding of the stomach walls and should not be used on a continuous basis. Acetaminophen (sold, among other brands, as Tylenol) has fewer side effects than Aspirin but its use beyond 10 days is discouraged without medical supervision. Antipyretics have been shown to act on the temperature-sensitive nerve cells in the preoptic or anterior hypothalamus of the brain. Among the painkillers, tranquilizers and fever reducers, the most promising seems to be Aminopyrene (marketed as Pyramidon). Taken orally, it enters the brain and other body tissues quite rapidly, with analgesic (pain killing) and antipyretic effects. In a comparative study of aminopyrene, the tranquilizer chlorpromazine and the painkiller sodium salicylate, all three caused a drop in temperature but only aminopyrene acted without affecting behavior or producing discomfort. The aminopyrene, at a dosage of 75 milligrams per kilogram of body weight, lowered body temperature about two degrees C with a duration of one to three hours. (It is made by the Aldrich Chemical Company as 4 dimethylaminoantipyrene.)

Aminopyrene, however, seems too short-lasting in the dosages tested as safe. Other temperature-lowering drugs include apomorphine, phenelzine, reserpine, levodopa, tetrodoxin, oxotremorine, sodium nitroprusside and THC. This last drug (Tetrahydrocannabinol) is an active part of hashish and yes, it is illegal in North America. THC (D9 variety) has been demonstrated to bring about a pronounced drop in body temperature with effects that proved to be both rapid in onset and prolonged in duration at the 50mg/kg dosage used. However, after three days the animals (mice) began to show reduced temperature-lowering effects and the dosage had to be increased by 20mg/kg to overcome this. Humans might not need a higher dosage for a month or more. But like even the best medications ever investigated, the drug effect doesn't last forever and more lasting interventions will have to be found.

Prednisolone, a growth-retarding compound, has been successfully used on mice to double their life span. It also is an antidepressant that can reduce aggression. Here again we have a substance, this time a legal one, that can raise the spirits, relax hostilities and slow the metabolism, resulting in long life. However, prednisolone inhibits the physical growth of the taker and is *not recommended* for children. With some imagination, however, we might visualize some pet shops stocking prednisolone-treated lion cubs ... happy, unaggressive, long-lived, and, like Peter Pan, resistant to growing up.

There may be other ways to slow metabolism without affecting body temperature. If we reduced our heart rate, for example, would aging respond accordingly? Animals such as elephants, whales or turtles, which have slow heart rates (six beats per minute), live longer than vertebrates with fast heart rates (mice: 600 beats per minute). Researchers at the University of Virginia's School of Medicine performed studies in which they chose 514 mice of both sexes and sequestered them in cages, putting ten mice in each cage. The control group was fed normally while the treated mice received a diet supplement of Lanoxin brand Digoxin (125mg/kg) to slow their heart rates. Having been treated from weaning to death, the treated males lived 30% longer, the females 13% longer. Both groups averaged equal amounts of food consumption, so caloric intake was not a factor. The last two survivors of the treated mice lasted beyond

Looking at the Thermometer

1,100 days, which is a significant record of life extension among mice. They might have lived longer still had it not been for the fact that at 1,120 days, Mouse No. 1 was decapitated by an escaped monkey and Mouse No. 2, the last survivor of this colony, was sacrificed for electron microscopic studies by the scientists. Such are the environmental hazards that effective survivors must contend with!

Earlier, McCay had noted that long-lived rats had heart rates averaging 20% per minute lower than normal. We therefore may conclude that a relaxed, slowed pulse seems to be an index of slowed aging, just as reduced core body temperature had been shown to be. As medications to slow the pulse rate have long been used to ease excessive tension, perhaps this approach could be used preventively as well.

Nutritional deficiencies in vitamin B6 or B5 (pantothenic acid) have been shown to lead to higher heat needs and raised core body temperature. Would the prolongevity dosage levels described in the previous chapter act preventively as well and keep the body temperature low?

What of the internal thermostat itself? What is it?

Body temperature is regulated by the activity of serotonin and noradrenalin on nerve cells in the anterior hypothalamus of the brain. Thermo-sensitive brain cells trigger body temperature directly through physiology and indirectly through behavior (e.g., shivering). This direct physiological control is based in the anteriorpreoptic hypothalamus while the indirect behavioral control is based in the posterior hypothalamus. The anterior (responsible for regulating adrenal and thyroid flow) senses and orders while the posterior (body control) acts. But the thermostat can be fooled. If it is warmed internally, body temperature lowers even if the animal is in a very cold room. However, peripheral senses can affect the thermostat as well. The pineal gland (our vestigial "third eye") influences body temperature regulation. It, in turn, is affected by cycles of light and time. Here physiology has traced a path for us right back to the environment: our life and its length, and our body and its temperature, continue to be reflections of what we surround ourselves with.

What other ways are there to reduce core body temperatures? People can develop fevers as a result of conflict, stress or psychogenic need. If that is so, then we might expect there to be a capacity of conscious or unconscious choice, that if we knew how to exercise it, could help us determine what our internal temperature should be. As David Cheek was successful in treating fever with hypnosis, perhaps self-hypnotic techniques could reset our brain's thermostat to a lower level. However, there is a built-in drawback to using hypnosis for lowering body temperature; for most hypnotic subjects, temperature increases as they move into the relaxed state. The effect is so reliable that it has been used as a hallmark of genuine hypnosis.

Successful personal growth or therapy can also lower the core body temperature. Primal therapy advocate Dr. Michael Holden observed that patients who had successfully undergone primal therapy looked more youthful, had a decreased pulse rate, lower blood pressure and reduced body temperature, as well as a slower brain wave amplitude on the EEG (electroencephalograph). He therefore hypothesized that since neurosis may be a speeded up (hyper) metabolic process resulting from the repressed pain of neonatal and childhood experience. Primal Therapy, when effective, could slow the rate of aging. The successful post-primal state required would have to be based on "connected primals" (insights as well as feelings) rather than solely on "abreacted primals" (feelings alone). Another study by Dr. Holden bases its conclusions on case history data that showed permanent change (lowered body temperature) had taken place for post-primal patients. He states:

> We are confronted by the fact that primal therapy lowers core body temperature in humans, presumably, by altering the intrinsic physiological mechanisms in the hypothalamus. The fact that this does occur challenges the notion that *37* degrees centigrade is truly the normal body temperature, genetically determined, for human beings.... The vital sign changes ... provide one with objective physiologic parameters to follow as an index of the therapeutic process and frees one from the obligation of following behavioral changes only.

Immunization has also been proposed as a technique for slowing the thermodynamic process. The assumption is that age-accelerating enzymes act as catalysts to precipitate the breakdown of key body proteins. A process advanced by two Texas researchers would isolate the offending human age-accelerators ("racemases") and inoculate a horse with them. The horse's immune system then would produce antibodies which could be extracted, purified, and concentrated for human use. The dosage would inhibit aging up to six months before another horse would need to be inoculated and bled. Of course, this process is still in the speculative stages and it is just as well. Who would want to raise racemase horses in Texas? People would think you were stuttering when you explained your mission to them and bleeding the animals could certainly get you shot.

Could it be that our healthiest core body temperature has always been about 88 degrees Fahrenheit and not 98.6? Have we gathered an average 10 degree deficit (or speeded up metabolism and shortened life span) from environmental stress and other detriments? Is our progress to correct psychological stress, self-induced and otherwise, measured by our body temperature?

On Sleep

When addressing groups interested in applied gerontology, someone from the audience is almost sure to ask: "How much sleep do we *really* need?" This question usually mobilizes the attention of the crowd and a wary professional will realize that many couples in the audience have spent up to 50 years hotly debating this issue. Taking sides will do little good. What I usually do is acknowledge the probable history of the debate. In the case of most couples, the partner who sleeps less than the other is often offended by the discrepancy, interpreting it as the other partner's laziness. Napoleon used to brag about needing very little sleep; consequently he sought out officers with the same rapid metabolic rate. At the turn of the century, our own continental culture heroes espoused the same sleep minima as "Nappy." Thomas Edison claimed to sleep not more than two hours a day, though his recent and more candid biographers claim he catnapped all day long in the lab. It is understandable that the cultural bias that associates sleep with laziness results in conflict concerning sleep. The brief sleeper may also be an insomniac who resents the partner's sound sleep, particularly if the partner's snores contribute to the insomnia. Another reason for conflict might be a basic philosophical intolerance for individual differences. My usual reply to the question, "what number of hours should we (all of us)

Growing Younger

sleep?" is that as people have varying metabolic rates and varying environmental stresses there is no one number of hours appropriate to us all. People should sleep until they are no longer tired, and I suggest we celebrate the differences or, at least, tolerate them.

Having said that, and seeing the crowd visibly relax, I do raise one concern. If someone consistently requires several hours more sleep than before, or if sleeping covers most of a 24-hour period for several days in succession, it might be a sign of reaction to stress or disease. The solution is not to remove the healing effects of sleep, but to seek the cause of the need for so much healing. If a medical checkup yields nothing, the psychological environment should be reviewed, probably by a professional counselor. Sleep time will automatically return to normal when the stressor departs. If this does not happen, we could expect increased sleep time to be paralleled by accelerated aging.

Sleep is the effect, not the cause, at least in the following examples. People who average more than 9 hours of sleep (or less than 6) per day have shorter life expectancies than those who average 6 to 8 hours per day. Too much sleep may be as bad for you as too little. Among those sleeping an average of 10 or more hours I would expect to find at least two factors at work. The main one would be a response to stress or body distress; help should be provided without curtailing the sleep as long as it is needed. Where no help is forthcoming, we would expect accelerated aging and a shortened lifespan. A second contributing factor that must not be missed would apply to those rare people with low blood pressure, slow metabolism, and low body temperature, who use sleep for a variety of purposes beyond physical rest. They enjoy their dreams and use them for psychological relief, healing, creativity and fun. For them, time acceleration (see Chapter 10) might be accomplished faster, but short of such a radical method, to curtail their sleep would be a mistake. For they are the slow aging minority, the one-in-six that is naturally age-resistant.

In general, you need enough sleep to feel rested and ready for a new day. If you think it takes you too long to reach that stage (especially if it is 12 hours or more), you might see if your life style or your health need to be improved.

Looking at the Thermometer

The following is an example of sleep as an anti-aging agent: In a lab experiment an old dog whose teeth had fallen out and whose coat had turned dull was kept asleep with "a harmless drug" for 23 out of every 24 hours for a period of 3 months. Under supervision of a staff of doctors and technicians, he received intravenous concentrations of vitamins, proteins and other food supplements "to accelerate metabolism and cellular growth." Presumably, in the hour he was awake, the dog relieved himself, was exercised and petted. After the sixth week, changes began to occur. His coat grew soft and glossy, and by the twelfth week, the end of the experiment, new teeth had begun to form and the animal seemed to have a puppy's energy. Finally, the doctors reported, "this rejuvenated canine fathered several litters of puppies during the next three years and might have for the second time reached old age had it not been killed while playing with a chimpanzee."

Of course, this anecdotal tale would need scientific replication. Although the intravenous diet may have made the difference, a similar test on a human would probably take 18 months (we live six times as long as dogs). I'll settle for replicating it on a dog first! An intriguing treatment, assuming sleep is central to rebuilding and rejuvenating the body.

Some Ideas on Metabolic Aging

Test your body age at the same time each day (temperature is cyclic for a variety of people). Make sure your temperature recording equipment is accurate.

Do different groups have different temperatures or temperature cycles?

What can *you* do to lower your body age (safely and legally) through lowering your temperature?

Are heart rate, EEG, or life-long growth rate related to body age?

Growing Younger

~7~
Looking
OUTSIDE OURSELVES
Altitude, Anthropology and Attitude

WE ALL ARE profoundly affected by our environment: its geography, its social and cultural expectations, and even its shape. Can aging itself be accelerated or slowed by the environment? We will examine the most recent evidence in three basic categories: altitude, anthropology and attitude.

Altitude
An analysis of United States counties shows that those with low annual death rates usually are situated at higher elevations than those with high death rates. Looking at their death statistics, we find that three states—Colorado, Wyoming and Utah—are at elevations higher than 6,000 feet, and have an average death rate of 81 per 10,000. The three lowest-lying states—Delaware, Louisiana, Florida—with 100 feet or less elevation, average 100 deaths per 10,000. The national death rate, was in 'the low 90s per 10,000 population.

If we look at longevity in terms of years, a similar pattern emerges. Demographic work in this connection, and its effect on cultures in which people expect to live past 100 (and usually do), has revealed that long-lived peoples tend to reside at altitudes of at least a mile above sea level.

Some researchers were skeptical about early demographic reports on these long-lived societies. They felt that many of the citizens interviewed were too old to possess formal birth certificates that could prove their ages. However, in subsequent volumes published by Sula Benet, an anthropologist at the Research Institute for the Study of Man in New York, documentation was more thorough

Growing Younger

and meticulous as she was able to consult church records and obtain other key family data. The past concern that such longevity claims are both unproved and unprovable is no longer tenable in the face of the anthropological and medical records reviewed by Dr. Benet.

Before we take a closer look at these long-lived cultures, let us explore why altitude might have such an important effect on aging.

Among people living at high altitudes there is higher oxygen-carrying capacity per unit volume of blood and a generally expanded blood volume. The lungs must work harder to carry the oxygen and the body must exert itself more in normal activity. For those adults who move to such regions at an advanced age this may be an initial disadvantage because much body adjustment must take place. But the bodies of individuals born in this environment are able to cope well with high altitude living. (In many areas of the world, race horses reared at altitudes greater than one mile are not allowed to take part in general competition with rivals from lower-lying regions.)

High-altitude communities also may benefit from cleaner air, greater isolation from technological stress, or the inherent need for more exercise to accomplish daily work. Furthermore, the effect of being relatively isolated by living in a setting that contains various built-in hardships may tend to foster more cooperative and therefore emotionally healthier attitudes among people. The advantages of this kind of social environment have even been demonstrated with animals.

Yet, for aging, there may be a limit to height advantage, and I would guess that an altitude between 5 and 10 thousand feet may be the ideal. However, we would need additional body age data and more general health information to confirm this.

Anthropology

We cannot attribute the effects of reduced aging to altitude alone. Long-lived societies undoubtedly exemplify many of the principles that gerontologists have discovered. However, we must examine the work of Sula Benet, who was among the first to pioneer the study of one of the longest-lived societies on earth today—the Abkhasians of the USSR'S Caucasus Mountains. Here are her observations:

Looking Outside Ourselves

WHY THEY LIVE TO BE 100, OR EVEN OLDER, IN ABKHASIA*

Not long ago, in the village of Tarnish in the Soviet Republic of Abkhasia, I raised my glass of wine to toast a man who looked no more than 70. "May you live as long as Moses (120)," I said. He was not pleased. He was 119.

For centuries, the Abkhasians and other Caucasian peasants have been mentioned in the chronicles of travelers amazed at their longevity and good health. Even now, on occasion, newspaper reports in the United States and elsewhere (never quite concealing bemusement and skepticism) will tell of an Abkhasian who claims to be 120, sometimes 130. When I returned from Abkhasia to New York displaying photographs and statistics, insisting that the tales are true and preoccupied with the question of why, my American friends invariably responded with the mocking question that contained its own answer: "Yogurt?" As a matter of fact, no not yogurt; but the Abkhasians do drink a lot of buttermilk.

Abkhasia is a hard land—the Abkhasians, expressing more pride than resentment, say it was one of God's afterthoughts— but it is a beautiful one; if the Abkhasians are right about its mythical origin, God had a good second thought. It is subtropical on its coast along the Black Sea, alpine if one travels straight back from the sea, through the populated lowlands and valleys, to the main range of the Caucasus Mountains.

The Abkhasians have been there for at least 1,000 years. For centuries they were herdsmen in the infertile land, but now the valleys and foothills are planted with tea and tobacco, and they draw their living largely from agriculture. There are 100,000 Abkhasians, not quite a fifth of the total population of the autonomous Abkhasian Republic, which is, administratively, part of Georgia, Joseph Stalin's birthplace; the rest are Russians, Greeks and Georgians.

---

*Dr Sula Benet's work reproduced here was originally published in the *New York Times,* December 26, 1971. © 1971 by the New York Times Company. Reprinted with permission.

Growing Younger

However, most of the people in government are Abkhasian, and both the official language and style of life throughout the region are Abkhasian. The single city, Sukhumi, is the seat of government and a port of call for ships carrying foreign tourists. They are often visible in the streets of the city, whose population includes relatively few Abkhasians. Even those who live and work there tend to consider the villages of their families their own real homes. It is in the villages—575 of them between the mountains and the sea ranging in population from a few hundred to a few thousand—that most Abkhasians live and work on collective farms.

I first went there in the summer of 1970 at the invitation of the Academy of Sciences of the USSR. The Abkhasians were fascinating; I returned last summer and will go again next year. It was while interviewing people who had participated in the early efforts at collectivization that I became aware of the unusually large number of people, ranging in age from 80 to 119, who are still very much a part of the collective life they helped organize.

After spending months with them, I still find it impossible to judge the age of older Abkhasians. Their general appearance does not provide a clue; you know they are old because of their gray hair and the lines on their faces, but are they 70 or 107? I would have guessed "70" for all of the old people that I encountered in Abkhasia, and most of the time I would have been wrong.

It is as if the physical and psychological changes which to us signify the aging process had, in the Abkhasians, simply stopped at a certain point. Most work regularly. They are still blessed with good eyesight, and most have their own teeth. Their posture is unusually erect, even into advanced age; many take walks of more than two miles a day and swim in the mountain streams. They look healthy, and they are a handsome people. Men show a fondness for enormous mustaches, and are slim but not frail. There is an old saying that when a man lies on his side, his waist should be so small that a dog can pass beneath it. The women are darkhaired and also slender, with fair complexions and shy smiles.

There are no current figures for the total number of aged in Abkhasia, though in the village of Dzhgerda, which I visited last summer, there were 71 men and 100 women between 81 and 96 and 19 people over 91—13 percent of the village population of 1,200.

Looking Outside Ourselves

And it is worth noting that this extraordinary percentage is not the result of a migration by the young. Abkhasians, young and old, understandably prefer to stay where they are, and rarely travel, let alone migrate. In 1954, the last year for which overall figures are available, 2.58 percent of the Abkhasians were over 90. The roughly comparable figures for the entire Soviet Union and the United States were 0.1 percent and 0.4 percent, respectively.

Since 1932, the longevity of the Abkhasians has been systematically studied on several occasions by Soviet and Abkhasian investigators, and I was given full access to their findings by the Ethnographic Institute in Sukhumi. These studies have shown that, in general, signs of arteriosclerosis, when they occurred at all, were found only in extreme old age. One researcher who examined a group of Abkhasians over 90 found that close to 40 percent of the men and 30 percent of the women had vision good enough to read or thread a needle without glasses, and that over 40 percent had reasonably good hearing. There were no reported cases of either mental illness or cancer in a nine-year study of 123 people over 100.

In that study, begun in 1960 by Dr. G.N. Sichinava of the Institute of Gerontology in Sukhumi, the aged showed extraordinary psychological and neurological stability. Most of them had clear recollection of the distant past, but partially bad recollection for more recent events. Some reversed this pattern, but quite a large number retained a good memory of both the recent and distant past. All correctly oriented themselves in time and place. All showed clear and logical thinking, and most correctly estimated their physical and mental capacities. They showed a lively interest in their families' affairs, in their collective and in social events. All were agile, neat and clean.

Abkhasians are hospitalized only rarely, except for stomach disorders and childbirth. According to doctors who have inspected their work, they are expert at setting broken arms and legs themselves—their centuries of horsemanship have given them both the need and the practice.

The Abkhasian view of the aging process is clear from their vocabulary. They do not have a phrase for "old people"; those over 100 are called "long living people." Death, in the Abkasian view, is not the logical end of life but something irrational. The aged seem to

Growing Younger

lose strength gradually, wither in size and finally die; when that happens, Abkhasians show their grief fully, even violently.

For the rest of the world, disbelief is the response not to Abkhasians' deaths but to how long they have lived. There really should no longer be any question about their longevity. All of the Soviet medical investigators took great care to crosscheck the information they received in interviews. Some of the men studied had served in the army, and military records invariably supported their own account. Extensive documentation is lacking only because the Abkhasians had no functioning written language until after the Russian Revolution.

But why do they live so long? The absence of a written history, and the relatively recent period in which medical and anthropological studies have taken place, preclude a clear answer. Genetic selectivity is an obvious possibility. Constant hand-to-hand combat during many centuries of Abkhasian existence may have eliminated those with poor eyesight, obesity and other physical shortcomings, producing healthier Abkhasians in each succeeding generation. But documentation for such an evolutionary process is lacking.

When I asked the Abkhasians themselves about their longevity, they told me that they live as long as they do because of their practices in sex, work and diet.

The Abkhasians, because they expect to live long and healthy lives, feel it is necessary self-discipline to conserve their energies, including their sexual energy, instead of grasping what sweetness is available to them at the moment. They say it is the norm that regular sexual relations do not begin before the age of 30 for men, the traditional age of marriage; it was once even considered unmanly for a new husband to exercise his sexual rights on his wedding night. (If they are asked what is done to provide substitute gratifications of normal sexual needs before marriage, Abkhasians smile and say, "Nothing," but it is not unreasonable to speculate that they, like everyone else, find substitutes for the satisfaction of healthy, heterosexual sex. Today, some young people marry in their mid-20s instead of waiting for the "proper" age of 30, to the consternation of their elders.)

Postponement of satisfaction may be smiled at, but so is the expectation of prolonged, future enjoyment, perhaps with more reason.

Looking Outside Ourselves

One medical team investigating the sex life of the Abkhasians concluded that many men retain their sexual potency long after the age of 70, and 13.6 percent of the women continue to menstruate after the age of 55.

Tarba Sit, 102, confided to me that he had waited until he was 60 to marry because while he was in the army "I had a good time right and left." At present, he said with some sadness, "I have a desire for my wife, but no strength." One of his relatives had nine children, the youngest born when he was 100. Doctors obtained sperm from him when he was 119, in 1965, and he still retained his libido and potency. The only occasion on which medical investigators found discrepancies in the claimed ages of Abkhasians was when men insisted they were younger than they actually were. One said he was 95, but his daughter had a birth certificate proving she was 81, and other information indicated he was really 108. When he was confronted with the conflict he became angry and refused to discuss it, since he was about to get married. Makhil Tarkil, 104, with whom I spoke in the village of Duripah, said the explanation was obvious in view of the impending marriage: "A man is a man until he is 100, you know what I mean. After that, well, he's getting old."

Abkhasian culture provides a dependent and secondary role for women; when they are young, their appearance is stressed, and when they are married, their service in the household is their major role. (As with other aspects of Abkhasian life, the period since the revolution has brought changes, and some women now work in the professions; but in the main, the traditions are still in force.) In the upbringing of a young woman, great care is taken to make her as beautiful as possible according to Abkhasian standards. In order to narrow her waist and keep her breasts small, she wears a leather corset around her chest and waist; the corset is permanently removed on her wedding night. Her complexion should be fair, her eyebrows thin; because a high forehead is also desirable, the hair over the brow is shaved and further growth is prevented through the application of bleaches and herbs. She should also be a good dancer.

Virginity is an absolute requirement for marriage. If a woman proves to have been previously deflowered, the groom has a perfect right to take her back to her family and have his marriage gifts returned. He always exercises that right, returning the bride and announcing to the family, "Take your dead one." And to him, as well as all other eligible men, she is dead; in Abkhasian society, she has been so dishonored by his rejection that it would be next to impossible to find a man to marry her. (Later on, however, she may be married off to an elderly widower or some other less desirable male from a distant village. When she is discovered, she is expected to name the guilty party. She usually picks the name of a man who has recently died, in order to prevent her family from taking revenge and beginning a blood feud.)

For both married and unmarried Abkhasians, extreme modesty is required at all times. There is an overwhelming feeling of uneasiness and shame over any public manifestation of sex, or even affection. A man may not touch his wife, sit down next to her or even talk to her in the presence of strangers. A woman's armpits are considered an erogenous zone and are never exposed, except to her husband.

A woman is a stranger, although a fully accepted one, in her husband's household. Her presence always carries the threat that her husband's loyalty to his family may be eroded by his passion for her. In the Abkhasian tradition, a woman may never change her dress nor bathe in the presence of her mother-in-law, and when an Abkhasian couple are alone in a room, they keep their voices low so that the husband's mother will not overhear them.

Despite the elaborate rules—perhaps, in part, because they are universally accepted—sex in Abkhasia is considered a good and pleasurable thing when it is strictly private. And, as difficult as it may be for the American mind to grasp, it is guiltless. It is not repressed or sublimated into work, art or religious mystical passion. It is not an evil to be driven from one's thoughts. It is a pleasure to be regulated for the sake of one's health—like a good wine.

An Abkhasian is never "retired," a status unknown in Abkhasian thinking. From the beginning of life until its end, he does what he is capable of doing because both he and those around him consider work vital to life. He makes the demands on himself that he can meet, and as those demands diminish with age, his status in the community nevertheless increases.

In his nine-year study of aged Abkhasians, Dr. Sichinava made a detailed examination of their work habits. One group included 62

Looking Outside Ourselves

men, most of whom had been working as peasants from the age of 11, and 45 women who, from the time of adolescence, had worked in the home and helped care for farm animals. Sichinava found that the work load had decreased considerably between the ages of 80 and 90 for 48 men, and between 90 and 100 for the rest. Among the women, 27 started doing less work between 80 and 90, and the others slowed down after 90. The few men who had been shepherds stopped following the herds up to the mountain meadows in spring and instead began tending farm animals, after the age of 90. The farmers began to work less land; many stopped plowing and lifting heavy loads, but continued weeding (despite the bending involved) and doing other tasks. Most of the women stopped helping in the fields and some began to do less housework.

Instead of serving the entire family—an Abkhasian family, extended through marriage, may include 50 or more people— they served only themselves and their children. But they also fed the chickens and knitted.

Dr. Sichinava also observed 21 men and 7 women over 100 years old and found that, on the average, they worked a four-hour day on the collective farm—the men weeding and helping with the corn crop, the women stringing tobacco leaves. Under the collective system, members of the community are free to work in their own gardens, but they get paid in what are, in effect, piecework rates for the work they do for the collective. Dr. Sichinava's group of villagers over 100, when they worked for the collective, maintained an hourly output that was not quite a fifth that of the norm for younger workers. But in maintaining their own pace, they worked more evenly and without wasted motion, stopping on occasion to rest. By contrast, the younger men worked rapidly, but competitively and tensely. Competitiveness in work is not indigenous to Abkhasian culture but it is encouraged by the Soviet Government for the sake of increased production; pictures of the best workers are posted in the offices of the village collectives. It is too soon to predict whether this seemingly fundamental change in work habits will affect Abkhasian longevity.

The persistent Abkhasians have their own workers' heroes: Kelkiliana Kheza, a woman of 109 in the village of Otapi, was paid for 49 workdays (a collective's workday is eight hours) during one summer; Pozba Pash, a man of 94 on the same collective, worked 155 days one year; Minoayan Grigorii of Aragich, often held up as an example to the young, worked 230 days in a year at the age of 90. (Most Americans, with a two-week vacation and several holidays, work between 240 and 250 days, some of them less than eight hours, in a year.)

Both the Soviet medical profession and the Abkhasians agree that their work habits have a great deal to do with their longevity. The doctors say that the way Abkhasians work helps the vital organs function optimally. The Abkhasians say, "Without rest, a man cannot work; without work, the rest does not give you any benefit."

That attitude, though it is not susceptible to medical measurements, may be as important as the work itself. It is part of a consistent life pattern. When they are children, they do what they are capable of doing, progressing from the easiest to the most strenuous tasks, and when they age, the curve descends, but it is unbroken. The aged are never seen sitting in chairs for long periods, passive like vegetables. They do what they can, and while some consider the piecework system of the collectives a form of exploitation, it does permit them to function at their own pace.

Overeating is considered dangerous in Abkhasia, and fat people are regarded as ill. When the aged see a younger Abkhasian who is even a little overweight, they inquire about his health. "An Abkhasian cannot get fat," they say. "Can you imagine the ridiculous figure one would cut on horseback?" But to the dismay of the elders, the young eat much more than their fathers and grandfathers do; light, muscular and agile horsemen are no longer needed as a first line of defense.

The Abkhasian diet, like the rest of life, is stable; investigators have found that people 100 years and older eat the same foods throughout their lives. They show few idiosyncratic preferences, and they do not significantly change their diet when their economic status improves. Their caloric intake is 23 percent lower than that of the industrial workers in Abkhasia, though they consume twice as much vitamin C; the industrial workers have a much higher rate of coronary insufficiency and a higher level of cholesterol in the blood.

The Abkhasians eat without haste and with decorum. When guests are present, each person in turn is toasted with praise of his

Looking Outside Ourselves

real or imaginary virtues. Such meals may last several hours, but nobody minds, since they prefer their food served lukewarm in any case. The food is cut into small pieces, served on platters, and eaten with the fingers. No matter what the occasion, Abkhasians take only small bites of food and chew those very slowly—a habit that stimulates the flow of ptyalin and maltase, insuring proper digestion of the carbohydrates which form the bulk of the diet. And, traditionally, there are no leftovers in Abkhasia; even the poor dispose of uneaten food by giving it to the animals, and no one would think of serving warmed-over food to a guest—even if it had been cooked only two hours earlier. Though some young people, perhaps influenced by Western ideas, consider the practice wasteful, most Abkhasians shun day-old food as unhealthful.

The Abkhasians eat relatively little meat—perhaps once or twice a week—and prefer chicken, beef, young goat and, in the winter, pork. They do not like fish, and despite its availability, rarely eat it. The meat is always freshly slaughtered and either broiled or boiled to the absolute minimum—until the blood stops running freely or, in the case of the chicken, until the meat turns white. It is, not surprisingly, tough in the mouth of a non-Abkhasian, but they have no trouble with it.

At all three meals, the Abkhasians eat abista, a corn meal mash cooked in water without salt, which takes the place of bread. Abista is eaten warm with pieces of homemade goat cheese tucked into it. They eat cheese daily, and also consume about two glasses of buttermilk a day. When eggs are eaten, which is not very often, they are boiled or fried with pieces of cheese.

The other staples in the Abkhasian diet—staple in Abkhasia means daily or almost so—include fresh fruits, especially grapes; fresh vegetables, including green onions, tomatoes, cucumbers and cabbage; a wide variety of pickled vegetables, and baby lima beans, cooked slowly for hours, mashed and served flavored with a sauce of onions, peppers, garlic, pomegranate juice and pepper. That hot sauce, or a variant of it, is set on the table in a separate dish for anyone who wants it. Large quantities of garlic are also always at hand.

Although they are the main suppliers of tobacco for the Soviet Union, few Abkhasians smoke. (I did meet one, a woman over 100, who smoked constantly.) They drink neither coffee nor tea. But they do consume a locally produced, dry, red wine of low alcoholic content. Everyone drinks it, almost always in small quantities, at lunch and supper, and the Abkhasians call it "life giving." Absent from their diet is sugar, though honey, a local product, is used. Toothaches are rare.

Soviet medical authorities who have examined the Abkhasians and their diet feel it may well add years to their lives; the buttermilk and pickled vegetables, and probably the wine, help destroy certain bacteria and indirectly prevent the development of arteriosclerosis, the doctors think. A team of Soviet doctors and Dr. Samuel Rosen of New York, a prominent ear surgeon, compared the hearing of Muscovites and Abkhasians, and concluded that the Abkhasians' diet— very little saturated fat, a great deal of fruit and vegetables— also accounted for their markedly better hearing. The hot sauce is the only item most doctors would probably say "no" to, and apparently some Abkhasians feel the same way.

Although the Abkhasians themselves attribute their longevity to their work, sex and dietary habits, there is another, broader aspect of their culture that impresses an outsider in their midst: the high degree of integration in their lives, the sense of group identity that gives each individual an unshaken feeling of personal security and continuity, and permits the Abkhasians as a people to adapt themselves—yet preserve themselves—to the changing conditions imposed by the larger society in which they live. That sense of continuity in both their personal and national lives is what anthropologists would call their spatial and temporal integration.

Their spatial integration is in their kinship structure. It is, literally, the Abkhasians' all-encompassing design for living: It regulates relationships between families, determines where they live, defines the position of women and marriage rules. Through centuries of nonexistent or ineffective centralized authority, kinship was life's frame of reference, and it still is.

Kinship in Abkhasia is an elaborate, complex set of relationships based on patrilineage. At its center is the family, extended through marriage by the sons; it also includes all those families which can be traced to a single progenitor; and, finally to all persons with the same surname, whether the progenitor can be traced or not. As a result, an Abkhasian may be "kin" to several thousand people, many of whom he does not know. I first discovered the pervasiveness of kinship rules when my friend, Omar, an Abkhasian who had accompanied me from Sukhumi to the village of Duripsh, introduced me to a number of people he called his brothers and sisters. When I had met more than 20 "siblings" I asked, "How many brothers and sisters do you have?"

"In this village, 30," he said. "Abkhasian reckoning is different from Russian. These people all carry my father's name."

I took his explanation less seriously than I should have. Later, when I expressed admiration for a recording of Abkhasian epic poetry I had heard in the home of one of Omar's "brothers," Omar, without a word, gave the record to me as a gift.

"Omar, it isn't yours," I said.

"Oh yes it is. This is the home of my brother," he said. When I appealed to the "brother," he said, "Of course he can give it to you. He is my brother."

The consanguineal and affinal relationships that make up the foundation of the kinship structure are supplemented by a variety of ritual relationships that involve lifetime obligations—and serve to broaden the human environment from which Abkhasians derive their extraordinary sense of security. Although there are no alternative lifestyles towards which the rebellious may flee, the Abkhasians are ready to absorb others into their own culture. During my visit, for instance, a Christian man was asked to be the godfather of a Moslem child; both prospective godfather and child were Abkhasians. When I expressed surprise, I was told, "It doesn't matter. We want to enlarge our circle of relatives."

The temporal integration of Abkhasian life is expressed in its general continuity, in the absence of limiting, defining conditions of existence like "unemployed," "adolescent," "alienated." Abkhasians are a life-loving, optimistic people, and unlike so many very old "dependent" people in the United States—who feel they are a burden to themselves and their families—they enjoy the prospect of continued life. One 99-year-old Abkhasian, Akhba Suleiman of the village of Achandara, told his doctor, "It isn't time to die yet. I am needed by my children and grandchildren, and it isn't bad in this world— except that I can't turn the earth over and it has become difficult to climb trees."

Growing Younger

The old are always active. "It is better to move without purpose than to sit still," they say. Before breakfast, they walk through the homestead's courtyard and orchard, taking care of small tasks that come to their attention. They look for fences and equipment in need of repair and check on the family's animals. At breakfast, their early morning survey completed, they report what has to be done.

Until evening, the old spend their time alternating work and rest. A man may pick up wind-fallen apples, then sit down on a bench, telling stories or making toys for his grandchildren or great-grandchildren. Another chore which is largely attended to by the old is weeding the courtyard, a large green belonging to the homestead, which serves as a center of activity for the kin group. Keeping it in shape requires considerable labor, yet I never saw a courtyard that was not tidy and well-trimmed.

During the summer, many old men spend two or three months high in the mountains, living in shepherds' huts helping to herd or hunting for themselves and the shepherds (with their arrested aging process, many are excellent marksmen despite their age). They obviously are not fearful of losing their authority during their absence; their time in the mountains is useful and pleasurable.

The extraordinary attitude of the Abkhasian—to feel needed at 99 or 110—is not an artificial, self-protective one; it is the natural expression, in old age, of a consistent outlook that begins in childhood. The stoic upbringing of an Abkhasian child, in which parents and senior relatives participate, instills respect, obedience and endurance. At an early age, children participate in household tasks; when they are not at school, they work in the fields or at home.

There are no separate "facts of life" for children and adults. The values given children are the ones adults live by, and there is no hypocritical disparity (as in so many other societies) between adult words and deeds. Since what they are taught is considered important, and the work they are given is considered necessary, children are neither restless nor rebellious. As they mature, there are easy transitions from one status in life to another; a bride, for instance, will stay for a time with her husband's relatives, gradually becoming part of a new clan, before moving into his home.

From the beginning, there is no gap between expectation and experience. Abkhasians expect a long and useful life and look for-

Looking Outside Ourselves

ward to old age with good reason; in a culture which so highly values continuity in its traditions, the old are indispensable in their transmission. The elders preside at important ceremonial occasions, they mediate disputes and their knowledge of farming is sought. They feel needed because, in their own minds and everyone else's, they are. They are the opposite of burdens; they are highly valued resources.

The Abkhasians themselves are obviously right in citing their diet and their work habits as contributing factors in their longevity; in my opinion, their postponed, and later prolonged, sex life probably has nothing to do with it. Their climate is exemplary, the air (especially to a New Yorker) refreshing, but it is not significantly different from many other areas of the world, where life spans are shorter. And while some kind of genetic selectivity may well have been at work, there simply is not enough information to evaluate the genetic factor in Abkhasian longevity....

The Abkhasians practice an elaborate folk medicine using more than 200 indigenous plants to cure a wide variety of ills. They apply plantain leaves to heal severe wounds, take ranaculuaes for measles, use poligonacese as an anticoagulant and amfetida (also known as Devil's Dung) as an antispasmodic. When all else fails, a doctor is called and the aged Abkhasian is taken to hospital—but always with the expectation, including his own, that he will recover. They never express the fatalistic view, "Well, what do you expect at that age?" Sickness is simply not considered normal and natural....

My own view is that Abkhasians live as long as they do primarily because of the extraordinary cultural factors that structure their existence; the uniformity and certainty of both individual and group behavior, the unbroken continuum of life's activities—the same games, the same work, the same food, the same self-imposed and socially perceived needs. And the increasing prestige that comes with increasing age.

There is no better way to comprehend the importance of these cultural factors than to consider for a moment some of the prevalent characteristics of American society. Children are sometimes given chores to keep them occupied, but they and their parents know there is no need for the work they do; even as adults, only a small percentage of Americans have the privilege of feeling that their work is essential and important. The old, when they do not simply vegetate, out of view and out of mind, keep themselves "busy" with bingo and shuffleboard. Americans are mobile, sometimes frantically so, searching for signs of performance that will indicate their lives are meaningful. Can Americans (western society) learn something from the Abkhasian view of "long living" people? I think so.

Half a decade after Sula Benet's original article appeared in the *New York Times,* her followup work was published in a book entitled *How to Live to be 100.* Dr. Benet has graciously granted us permission to reprint excerpts from this book so that we might follow the progress of the Abkhasians from a later perspective.

*A VISIT WITH THE OLDEST WOMAN IN THE WORLD**

Adding years to life i~ now not as important as adding life to years.
—SOVIET GERONTOLOGIST DAVYDOVSKII

It may be difficult to believe, but I have had the pleasure of meeting and knowing a delightful woman 139 years old. Khfaf Lazuria, according to the official register of her native village of Kutol, Abkhasia, was born on October 18, 1835;—in 1974, she was perhaps the oldest woman alive. I was taken to visit Khfaf by her grandnephew, Mushni Taevich, an eminent Abkhasian poet, who drove me to Kutol early one summer morning. We found Khfaf sitting comfortably in the shade of a large tree in the courtyard of her home. The courtyard was broad and spacious, covered with smooth green grass which was kept neat and trim not with a lawn-mower, but by the numerous animals—chickens, geese, turkeys, goats, and horses—which roamed and grazed freely.

---

*Reprinted from *How to Live to be 100* by Sula Benet (New York: Dial, 1976) © Sula Benet: reproduced with permission.

Looking Outside Ourselves

Although she had not been told of our coming, Khfaf was clearly delighted to have visitors, especially her favorite grand-nephew. She kissed Mushni and immediately asked him for a cigarette. Most Abkhasians do not smoke or drink hard liquor, but this breezy lady of 139 took great pleasure in puffing on the cigarette. After warm greetings and introductions, we sat down and I began to question her. Although her Russian was limited, she understood everything I asked, and we communicated with great ease.

She was quite small. I was told that she had been taller, but had seemed to have shrunk with the years. She was about five feet tall and like most Abkhasians, slender. Her face was astonishingly smooth with few wrinkles. Her eyes were bright, curious, alive—and often full of mischief. She had a keen sense of humor and laughed easily. She responded warmly to me, kissing my cheeks as an expression of her approval. When I returned her kiss, I noticed her fresh smell, like that of a young girl. She wore a simple, blue-and-white flowered dress made like a caftan. I could see that it had been washed many times, but was spotless and neat. A white polka-dotted cotton kerchief was wrapped around her head, and she wore pink slippers over gray stockings.

I told her I'd heard she could thread a needle without wearing glasses. She laughed. "I never had eyeglasses," she said. Would she do it for me? "Oh, yes! But we are sitting in the shade, so it must be white thread." Her great-granddaughter went into the house and brought out a needle and thread. Khfaf's agile fingers threaded the needle in just a few seconds. She held it up with a flourish. I'd prepared my camera to photograph the actual threading—an astonishing feat in itself—but she was so quick that I captured only her triumphant look as she pulled the thread through.

I asked whether her parents, too, had lived long. She said that her great-grandfather, Dzhadash, had lived to 160, and his grandson, Naruk, to 120. Her mother had also lived long. Khfaf remarked that "mother did not know how to get old," and that her first cousin, Bzhenia, lived to be 146. Khfaf had two brothers and three sisters, some of whom had died when they were "only" 90 or so, because of an epidemic. It's apparent that longevity does, indeed, run in her family. Her relatives later supported this fact.

Growing Younger

Her smile clearly revealed some remaining teeth, but I did not have the heart to ask her how many.

I asked for a toilet and one of the young schoolgirls accompanied me to the outhouse, which was at least five city blocks away from where we were sitting. (It is customary to place the outhouses some distance from the houses.) The girl remarked, "Khfaf uses the meadow over there because there is no odor." Further along, we came to a brook with a bench placed very close to it and a pail nearby. Khfaf bathed from the pail every morning, sprinkling herself with this lovely fresh water which she preferred to tap water. Despite the fact that she had caught a cold on a chilly day the year before, she was not discouraged from this routine.

Khfaf claimed that was the only cold she ever had, that measles had been her only childhood disease, and that her health was perfect. I asked her to what she attributes her good health. She told me she eats regularly. She always carried food with her on any long trip so that she could have her meals on time. She preferred eating small quantities frequently, rather than large meals.

Khfaf urged me to accept a cigarette from her grandnephew. When I declined, she told me that she herself had not smoked at all until she was a hundred. When her work in the collective fields slowed down and she spent more time at home, she had been bored and taken up smoking; actually, she smoked only occasionally—when someone offered her a cigarette. My guess is that, even more than smoking itself, she enjoyed the jaunty look it gave her. Indeed, she asked for a cigarette when she was about to be photographed.

She used to love horseback riding, but gave it up when she was about 100 because there were too many cars on the road, which frightened the horses. "By the way," she joked, "how about sending me a car to drive?" She laughed and everybody there joined in the laughter.

In her younger days, in addition to working in the collective fields, she was a well-known midwife. She announced proudly that she had brought more than a hundred babies into the world.

We were expecting another guest. Mushni referred to her as the "girl Khfaf married off." To my great surprise, the "girl" turned out to be almost a century old. Khfaf looked hardly older than this woman, Adusha Lazuria, who is happily married to a relative of Khfaf's. She was seventeen when Khfaf made the match.

Looking Outside Ourselves

We spent a few hours chatting. People came and went, refreshments were served, songs were sung, and Khfaf's stepson delighted me with a demonstration of national dancing. Then the whole household, including the stepson's daughter-in-law and her children, set up a table in the courtyard. It was a lovely day, not too hot. The usual fare appeared on the table: abista (cornmeal), chicken, boiled meat from a freshly slaughtered calf, fruit, and abundant wine for drinking and toasting. The young girls stood by with pitchers of wine ready to replenish everyone's glass. Khfaf rose and led me by the hand to the table where she seated me beside her. As the oldest, she presided over the table. To my astonishment, she had two vodkas and kept urging me to drink my wine. She was amazed when I declined the vodka.

Although I knew in a general way the intricate banquet ritual of speeches and toasting, and who must drink standing and who may remain seated, I wasn't completely clear on all the minute details. Khfaf was. She needed no prompting. I was asked to get up only once, when Khfaf made a speech in my honor.

The food was plentiful, but no one overindulged. As the hours passed in drinking, eating and talking, Khfaf showed no sign of fatigue. I, on the other hand, beginning to feel a bit tired, absentmindedly lowered my corn-on-the-cob to my lap. Suddenly I felt something and looked down to see two chickens boldly pecking away at my corn!

What struck me most about Khfaf and about all the long-lived people I was to come to know so well in the many regions of the Caucasus was the fullness of their humanity. Khfaf was interested in everything and thoroughly feminine, wearing silver rings on both hands, and examining my jewelry. She noticed a bit of lace on my petticoat and wanted to see more of it. She was a striking contrast to the "old" people in our own country, who have so often given up on life in their sixties. The idea that she should cease to have interests, desires, or feelings because she had reached a certain age would have been incomprehensible to her, or laughable.

Khfaf claimed that in her youth she never met an Abkhasian who could read or write. She herself remained illiterate, although she was fully aware that today things are very different and that everyone goes to school. Her grandnephew is a fine poet who translated

Growing Younger

Pushkin's *Eugene Onegin* into Abkhasian. She did not know Pushkin, but she understood what poetry is because she knew Abkhasian folksongs and ballads.

It is awesome to think of how much history her life-span embraced. In 1853, during the Crimean War, Khfaf was a young girl with thick braids who was taken away from Abkhasia in a Turkish boat. She did not return to her homeland until ten years later.

She married at the age of forty and gave birth to a son, but soon lost both son and husband. At fifty she married a Christian and was baptized; she was born a Muslim. Khfaf was a firm believer in marriage. Her fourth and last marriage took place in 1944 when she was 108. Recently Khfaf, concerned that her granddaughter-in-law's brother was still a bachelor, told him that it was silly not to be married and that if she had an offer she would most certainly marry again!

She was eighty-five years old in 1921 when Soviet power was established in Abkhasia. She helped to organize the first collective farm. When a new crop, tea, was introduced on the collective, she became a member of the first "tea brigade." In 1940 she traveled to Moscow for the first All-Union Agricultural Exhibition. At that time she was already 104 years old.

At the age of 128 she continued to work. During tea-harvesting time she could gather as much as twenty-five kilos a day. Her quickness and skill served as a model to other workers who learned from her how to do the job more easily.

In the Soviet village register of Kutol, under the number 469, Khfaf is listed as the head of the household although she was illiterate and extremely old. Living in Khfaf's compound, beside her stepson Tarkuk, a widower, are his youngest son, thirty-three, his wife, and their two children. The son works as a teacher at the collective.

Everyone respected and liked Khfaf. She played with the great-grandchildren, swept the large courtyard daily, took complete care of a good-size vegetable garden, and saw to all of her own needs, including her own laundry. The great respect given to old people precludes depriving them of any activity they choose to take part in. It is assumed that people of any age may participate fully in the life of the household—its duties and its pleasures.

Looking Outside Ourselves

Khfaf was not unique in the Caucasus, or even an oddity. Although the marvel of her longevity and vigor is enough in itself to delight and interest us, she was a relatively common phenomenon among the people of her region.

One day a friend called me. "Turn on your TV," said she. "Khfaf Lazuria is on." I rushed to the set but saw only the last part of Khfaf's one-hundred-fortieth birthday celebration. A delegation from Moscow had come with good wishes for Khfaf and TV cameras were there to film the occasion. Khfaf was asked to dance. She obliged. Shifting her cane from right hand to left, she alternately waved her arms as the style of the dance required. I don't think she really needed the cane to support herself. But a cane is a sign of respectability and dignity. After ninety, no one would think of being without a cane although for some it is more a nuisance than a help.

On a very cold day in autumn, Khfaf Lazuria, faithful to her custom, took her daily bath in the mountain stream. The next day she had a fever, and finally had to admit that she did not feel well. After two weeks, she asked her family to accompany her to the family cemetery which was about a city block away. She wished to select her burial place. She pointed to the grave of her husband. "There," she said, "I have no right to be buried because I was his second wife and I will not see him in the next world. His first wife is buried next to him and she will be with him in the next world. I would like to be buried here .. ." and she pointed to a place a bit higher—a lovely spot overlooking a meadow filled with flowers. She died on February 14, 1975.

I learned of her death from television, radio, and press reports. A month later I was able to visit her family. How different it was from my visit of a few months before. The family was subdued and quiet in her absence, and the house seemed bare and empty without her.

Her granddaughter-in-law took me to the cemetery. We had to climb a rather high fence in order to get there and I wondered silently how Khfaf had managed it. Before the fence, the young woman smiled, observing my hesitation. "Khfaf," she said, "used to come this way twice a day, saying that it would soon be her next home." Well, I am a pretty agile climber, with good balance, and I found that fence rather difficult to manage. And Khfaf did it twice a day every day before she died!

Growing Younger

A small wooden structure resembling a hut covered the grave, but it was open enough for me to see inside. There, a small table held a pitcher of water with a glass, and close by lay a package of cigarettes and matches, for Khfaf's use. It was strange to observe this pagan tradition, which the family felt was completely fitting, harmoniously merged with Christian burial rites. Back at the house, I was shown a room upstairs where a table had been prepared, displaying photographs of Khfaf at various stages of her life, lit by a candle like a shrine.

My involvement in the study of Khfaf and her people has its own history, with roots that reach deep into my early memories. As a child, I lived in Warsaw, Poland. My father made frequent business trips to the Caucasus and my mother often went there to "take the waters." They returned with colorful stories of the wonderful people with whom they had become friends in that land of towering mountains, plunging ravines, and remote villages. They promised to take me there someday and I yearned to go, but it was not to be—then.

My imagination had been firmly captured and my interest persisted, nonetheless. I read everything I could find in history and fiction about the land and its people. And the literature was abundant. Despite the fierce conflict between Russia and those Caucasians who resisted annexation, Russian writers of the second half of the nineteenth century celebrated the Caucasus lyrically. Pushkin, Lermontov, and Tolstoy found these proud people a source of inspiration.

Many years later, when I was grown and living on another continent, many miles from those enchanted mountains, the childhood dream curiously became a reality. It happened by chance and not by my design. As a professor of anthropology at Hunter College in New York, I had been asked to translate and edit for Doubleday & Co. an ethnographic study of a small Russian village. The study had been published originally by the Ethnographic Institute of the Academy of Science in Moscow. One fine spring day in 1970, after my translation had been published, I received a cable from the Academy officially inviting me to do ethnographic field work in Abkhasia. I hardly remembered where it was, except that it was in the Caucasus, and that was all I needed. Without stopping even to look at a map, I went straight to the telegraph office and sent a return cable to the Academy: "Thank you. Coming."

Looking Outside Ourselves

There was something so utterly right and fitting about such a study. I could hardly believe my good fortune. To be able to visit the land of my childhood fantasies, not as a tourist, but doing my chosen life work—as an anthropologist, to observe and record the daily lives of its people, and to share what I found there with others—what luck! It was as if things had come full circle for me and I could hardly wait for the school term to end so that I could get started. The time was spent in learning all I could about the people to whom I was going—and whom I had visited so many times in my imagination.

During that field trip, in which I conducted studies on the early collectivization of the villages, the people I interviewed kept referring me to older people who, they said, would know more than they did, since collectivization had taken place some forty years before. These old people did indeed remember the earliest times. I found myself interviewing an unusually large number of people who ranged in age from 80 to 110, all of whom were still active in village life.

They talked easily with me, answering a great number of questions, and expressed opinions on the advantages and disadvantages of a collective economy. I was especially impressed by their cheerfulness, vigor, and humor, and made many friends among them. Their lives, their work, and their important roles in the village were indeed fascinating, but beyond that, I grew increasingly interested in learning *why* they lived so long, and in such apparent health, good spirits, and productivity.

Since earliest antiquity, the Caucasian peoples have been known for their legendary longevity. Ancient Greek, Iranian, and Arabian chronicles attest amply to the existence of long-living peoples throughout the region. The latest Soviet census reported that 70 percent of all people reaching 110 years or more live in the Caucasian republics; the remaining 30 percent are found in all the territories of European Russia, Siberia, the Ukraine, Central Asia, and Kazakhstan.

There was nothing new in the *fact* of the Caucasians' longevity. What I wanted to discover was the reason for it. I was often tempted to ask them how they got to be so old, but felt it would have been in poor taste. Sometimes, however, they themselves would volunteer the answer: "I live the right way," they would say proudly. But what was the right way?

101

Growing Younger

In an effort to find answers to this complex question, I have returned six more times to the Caucasus between the summer of 1970 and the spring of 1975. Like all field work, it was not always easy, and sometimes quite difficult, especially in winter when mountain roads were icy and in some places impassable. Nestled between high-rising mountains, many villages are isolated from the outside world except for narrow paths, negotiable only in summer and only by experienced climbers. From the steep mountainsides above, the gigantic white tongues of glaciers descend almost to the edge of the villages. But it was important to see the people in all seasons, to see how they adapted their work and activities to seasonal changes.

I was fortunate to be able to speak fluent Russian, so that we could communicate directly, without translators. It is assumed outside the Soviet Union that all Caucasians are Russians. This is a misconception and, unfortunately, a widespread one. Although Russian is the official language and mandatory in the schools, and there are sizable Russian populations in many Caucasian cities, the Caucasus is a geographical area made up of many different republics and autonomous areas, such as Georgia, Azerbaijan, Abkhasia, Armenia, Daghestan, and scores of others, large and small. Each of the many groups speaks and writes its own language and keeps its own customs and traditions, although Russian is used for communication between the different republics and the central government.

The Caucasian people live not only a long time, but in health and strength. Soviet scientists have found few if any cases of the degenerative diseases which plague the United States and Russia proper, such as heart disease, arteriosclerosis, kidney stones, gall stones, coronary occlusion, and hypertension.

An Azerbaijanian gerontologist, Dr. Makhty Sultanov, observed a 117-year-old man in Kabardino-Balkaria who splits and saws logs for his hearth routinely. I was told by Said, a Caucasian ethnographer, of a man of ninety in the village of Kurchaloi, who lifted a ram by the scruff of the neck just to show that "he was still a man." This same ethnographer told of a 120-year-old man who married a woman of forty and fathered three children.

Numerous Soviet medical teams have researched, observed, and documented many similar facts. I myself saw old people in the Caucasus riding horses, weeding vigorously, swimming, presiding

Looking Outside Ourselves

over feast tables, participating in all the activities of family and community life, with no signs of exhaustion or fatigue. It seemed quite natural that Makhty Tarkil, a strikingly handsome, tall Abkhasian of 104, during a banquet his family gave in my honor, frequently patted my hand, offered to give me a fine horse as a gift, and generally behaved like a courting gentleman. It was inconceivable that men or women there, no matter how old, could think of themselves as merely existing, marking time waiting for death, unloved, unwanted, and useless. These old men and women would not think of missing the village competition in horseracing.

What a contrast to our American "senior citizens" in their sixties and seventies! Here, in the richest, most technologically advanced country in the world, older people are farmed out, discarded, hidden away in hospitals, nursing "homes," artificial retirement villages, or falsely cheerful apartment compounds. Tobe old means to be exiled from the active life of society.

In American culture, the individual loses value as he ages. He is considered a worn-out model by his employer, an old car to be traded in. He is treated more and more like a minor by his family. Once having attained maturity, brief as it is in American society, he is automatically on the road back to infantilism. His teen-age children inform him, in increasingly less subtle ways, that he is "old-fashioned" and unable to adapt to changing conditions. He is "over thirty" and untrustworthy. As he gets older, he is treated as increasingly forgetful, irresponsible, outdated, and outdistanced, and in keeping with this treatment, he begins to conform to expectations—we react as we are treated. Responsibility is taken from him, and in the "second childhood" he is thought to be fit only for childish games, like shuffleboard. He reacts by becoming infantile, making petty demands, being ill-tempered and unreasonable. He seems to want to return to "the good old days," which really means the period when he was considered a responsible adult.

The old in America envy the young, since the young are the center of all ongoing life. The young in turn look at the old with scorn and an air of superiority, feeling that they know everything and their parents are too old and conservative to grasp the changes in the world. Tension permeates the relations between the generations—the old try to keep up with the young, just as the middle class competes with the upper class and the poor try to climb into the middle class. In a society in which people are in constant competition, as individuals and in social groups, there is little relaxation or enjoyment.

Modern society creates a higher standard of living and at the same time makes greater demands on human psychological and biological organization, often disturbing or destroying the physical environment in the process. This has a double effect, both positive and negative, on longevity. While creating the objective hygienic and material conditions for the prolongation of life, it destroys traditional family structure, depriving the elderly of the emotional support of their relatives and of the feeling of being needed, thus counteracting the positive effects of the higher material standard of living.

Caucasian culture, admittedly, represents an older, more stable system, with minimal industrialization and technological change—hardly comparable structurally or economically. Nonetheless, the integrated culture of the Caucasus, where all age groups and social classes live in symbiosis and cooperation to the mutual advantage of all concerned, has much to teach modern industrial society, which for all its technology and higher material standard of living has not improved the quality of life nor met the basic social needs of humans of any age. A person, modern society has once again realized, is not infinitely plastic, but has psychological, biological, and social needs which demand attention and satisfaction. Any material or technological system which fails to take these needs into consideration is doomed to self-destruction.

Twenty-five percent of our current 210 million population is now over the age of sixty; this represents 52.5 million people. About 8 million people are seventy-five or over. The increased longevity of our population is going to have a tremendous impact on all aspects of society. It behooves us to take a long, hard look at societies where old age is graceful, harmonious, and productive.

Since the 1930s, Soviet scientists, in local gerontological institutes, have been studying the aged of the Caucasus medically and demographically. The Institute of Gerontology in Kiev, which is the center for gerontological studies, coordinates the findings of the local institutes. I had ample opportunity to discuss longevity with sci-

Looking Outside Ourselves

entists and medical personnel at the various centers. They were most generous in permitting me to see their unpublished research as well as their published articles. I benefited greatly from their experience, but medical research, as important as it is, could not answer the question of why we find this great concentration of longevity in the Caucasus and not, for instance, in Russia proper or in the Ukraine. Neither could medical research answer the question of how the Caucasians preserved their faculties....

Sula Benet's work provides substantial evidence that certain lifestyles contribute to greater longevity; ultimately, perhaps, for us all. Born in 1903, she epitomizes youthfulness, not only to Abkhasians appearing to age at half our rate, but to her own society as well. When I last spoke to her on the telephone she had just returned from the ski slopes. Her work continues at New York's Research Institute for the Study of Man. By her example she proceeds to exemplify success, banishing the specter of forced retirement.

Alexander Leaf, a professor of clinical medicine at Harvard Medical School and Chief of Medical Services at Massachusetts General Hospital was aware of Sula Benet's accounts of the Abkhasians, the Villacambans of Ecuador and the Hunzas of Kashmir in Pakistan. He decided to see all three regions for himself, and through direct examination and interviews, check the validity and rationale of longevity in these cultures.

Although he learned much from these cultures, he could not come up with a single formula to explain the extended youthfulness of their people. He stated that:

> We need to develop hobbies and interests which will provide for us a useful, enjoyable role compatible with our perception of ourselves and which sustains our status within our peer group. As leisure time increases we must develop such activities for our early as well as our late years. Society and government will have to yield considerably to help meet these psychological needs of the elderly in a supportive manner. A long life is worth living only if there is something worth living for.

No one in the three long-living communities Leaf visited practiced all the aspects we would identify as contributing to longevity.

Growing Younger

Nor, as he told us, was there any one clearly dominating secret of longevity. The high-altitude cultures showed a combination of several factors that seem essential to slower aging. Leaf asserted that although the residents of these cultures demonstrate a net lifestyle advantage over the rest of the contemporary world, a culture that practices all that we know about slowing the aging process (and that avoids all we have found to accelerate it) has not yet been found. We may have to build it ourselves.

Attitude

The main conclusion to be drawn from Benet's as well as Leaf's work is that our medicine, and our culture generally, must shift from their near-total preoccupation with curing illness to a more preventive approach, geared to building the health of those who are well. Anti-aging intervention must be applied before the body age reaches a disabling level. This is why we speak primarily to those under 70, although we cannot forget the plight of those over it.

Seventy years of body age, as we have seen in the field studies of Benet and Leaf, is not necessarily close at all to 70 years of chronological age. In Abkhasia, one is still young at 30 (and, I would guess, the body age, if assessed, would reflect that youth). But a person's attitude, developed within the context of family and cultural expectations, should not be ignored in these studies. We have seen that one can create a self-fulfilling prophecy about one's own length of life and rate of aging.

We choose our life much as we choose our death. The attitude conducive to slowed aging would be double-barreled, consisting of expectations of a long, youthful life, a feeling of satisfaction and a joy to live it. Remember that a positive view of life is a predictor of a greater survival potential; people who enjoy life stay with it longer. Measured body age is significantly lower for those who tell us they have been happy throughout their lives (but not for those saying happiness was recent). Chronic happiness, besides being related to low body age, good health, and a young (under 36) mother at one's birth, is significantly related to an above-average level of sexual activity, a conviction that most people are more good than bad, a feeling that life has been fair (and even the habit of squeezing toothpaste tubes rather than rolling them!).

Looking Outside Ourselves

What about chronic unhappiness? How does it affect aging? Depression is the number one mental health problem of the post-retirement generation. Being "old" in our society usually is to be in a state of acute stress; the self-concepts of health, usefulness, the future, sex, love, survival, time, and energy are often very low. Hans Selye, the father of stress theories, has devoted a lifetime to writing, researching and discussing just how debilitating stress can be. Successful approaches to acute and even chronic depression will be potent anti-aging ammunition.

Certainly, the field of psychosomatic medicine is experiencing a boom in the face of new research. Almost a century has passed since Freud amazed society by curing patients with conversation alone. Today, we are finally applying the concept of the unity of mind and body to alleviate our real killers: cancer, heart disease, etc. Bottled-up anger and chronic depression may trigger many of these killers; some would say that all diseases plaguing our partners on this planet are triggered by them. Psychotherapy, hypnosis, guided fantasy, drug therapy and lifestyle restructuring all affect aging, because all affect destructive life attitudes.

What can be done preventively? How can we promote a happy life from the start? We may have to begin from the point of conception. The mother should be young in body age and psychologically ready for her child. Destructive pollutants, prescription drugs and poor diet must be kept away from the growing fetus. The delicate cortical development in the first three months is crucial here: tranquilizers, coffee, cigarettes, benzedrine, LSD and damaging stress must be avoided at all costs. The mother and father must want the child and create a loving environment during the gestation period. At birth, the child already should have experienced several months of hearing good music and calm voice communication between its parents; auditory and memory capacity is present long before birth. LeBoyer advocates, by his "birth without violence" method, that delivery should be both painless and pleasant for the child. As it establishes from the outset a positive expectation of life that will be self-fulfilling, it is highly recommended. Follow-ups of the more than 1,000 babies born in this way find them to have become happy and positive children, who rarely cry. The oldest, however, were only 8 years old at the time they were studied; we will have to wait a bit longer to see whether these attitudes will last throughout adult life.

Growing Younger

Prevention of destructive life attitudes is also possible for adults, of any age. Perhaps the best example is the SAGE project begun in Berkeley, California by psychologist Gay Luce. Through a variety of techniques—from meditation to exercise to biofeedback—an attitude can emerge whereby a person of advanced years can still refuse to be old, scared, pushed around, or told "you're too old" or "you can't do anything." Some over 80 senior citizens can even renew their interest in romance and sex, for with increased success in physical functioning comes better emotional health, more self confidence and added pleasure in life.

Yet, all this is enough to appall those so accustomed to the status quo that they are afraid some people may be actually enjoying themselves. In this connection I recall an experience I had 16 years ago as a psychology student and volunteer subject in a project at Michigan State University. My friend Tom and I were asked, one at a time, to use a pursuit rotor machine and to report to the instructor as soon as we felt fatigue. At this point we would be requested to fill out a questionnaire. We also were told that we would fatigue quickly; in fact, in a matter of seconds. Before Tom and I began the experiment we had a free night to discuss it. As we were receiving course credits for participating, we felt that we were expected to be critical. Clearly, we felt, the perceptionist running the studies was not taking into account the subject's self-fulfilling prophecy to accept the statement, "You will fatigue in seconds." Therefore, Tom and I resolved to set ourselves in the opposite direction: "I will not fatigue at all ... ever." In that way, we thought, we would be an inspiration to our class.

The next morning, having stepped up to the pursuit rotor, I had to follow, with a metal rod, a metal disc wobbling around a turntable. Time on target was recorded. The words "You will fatigue in seconds" were repeated to me as I began. At the end of the class, three hours later, I was still going strong, *without fatigue,* and enjoying myself.

Subsequently, however, I was dropped as a subject because the instructor felt that my attitude was poor. The following week, it was Tom's turn. After working on the machine all day, he finally quit at dinner time, emerging from the test room to an applauding group of classmates. The instructor, however, was "underwhelmed" and told

Looking Outside Ourselves

both of us privately that if our performance "continued to show results significantly worse than those of our classmates," it would reflect on our grades. The next week, just before class, Tom and I had coffee with our colleagues. Rather than sharing our dilemma with them, Tom announced that he discovered the REAL meaning of the study: "They think your time before fatigue is correlated with your sexual potency."

That morning, our instructor chose as Subject No. 3 the eldest student in the class, an 83-year-old retired nurse. She stayed with the rotor, without fatigue, all day long, even arguing with the person who tried to turn it off. Her attitude proved most productive for us. As a result, the experiment was scrapped and the instructor soon left for a remote post ...

Some Ideas About Attitude and Altitude
What cultural attitudes about aging did you grow up with? What about the present? How would you change them? How would that affect your age?

If people born and raised at high altitudes age more slowly than those raised at low altitudes, how do crossovers affect aging?

Would a vacation in the mountains affect aging differently than a vacation at a beach resort at sea level? Is there an altitude so high it could hurt aging?

Are there significantly short-lived cultures you could investigate?

How do you react to stress? Do you bottle it up? See whether characteristic ways of dealing with frustration affect aging.

Growing Younger

~8~
Looking
BEYOND PRECONCEPTIONS
The Human Potentials Movement and Transpersonal Aging

OUR SHARED CONCEPT of reality naturally limits imagination. Yet both are part of our conscious experience, culturally shaped, and continuously evolving.

Potentials refer neither to the past nor to the present. Not impeded by what is or what has been, they describe what might be. Similarly, the human potentials movement refers to our individual and collective futures: wherever (and whatever) you are, growing begins from there.

Historically (but not too many years ago), humanistic or "Third Force" psychology was a reaction to the more entrenched schools of Behaviorism and Psychoanalysis. With a more optimistic view of the human future, the Third Force became extremely eclectic in its membership, points of view and areas of interest.

The definition of Third Force—based in large part, initially on what it *wasn't* (behavioristic or psychoanalytic)—took some time to separate into identifiable components. Eventually, strong factions of humanistic or existential persuasion emerged. The humanists sought out the techniques of self-actualized growth and development most likely to lead to human happiness; existentialists focused on issues of will, responsibility and awareness. Out of this dialectic came one group, perhaps the most focused of all on enhancing human potentials and maximizing personal growth: the transpersonal psychologists.

Chronologically, the transpersonal psychology movement is still young, a mere teenager. Along with a formal international asso-

Growing Younger

ciation, the *Journal of Transpersonal Psychology* was founded in 1969. As late as 1976, it defined its purpose as being concerned with: "metaneeds, transpersonal values and states, unitive consciousness, peak experiences, ecstasy, mystical experience, being essence, bliss, awe, wonder, self-actualization, transcendence of self, spirit, sacralization of everyday life, oneness, cosmic awareness, cosmic play, individual and species-wide synergy, the theories and practices of meditation, spiritual paths, transpersonal actualization, compassion; and related concepts, experiences, and activities."

Collectively, these grand if somewhat vague terms are a mixed blessing. Science and mysticism do not often blend easily; the heavy jargon promises much but delivers little. However, the major draw of this approach remains intact: after the drama is over, it explores rather successfully the most promising methods for upgrading human ability. Under the umbrella of transpersonal psychology one might include biofeedback, altered states of consciousness, innovative marriage and family patterns, accelerated and specialized education, hypnosis and auto-hypnosis, as well as the contemporary emphasis on holistic health or the primary prevention of serious human problems. Despite the occasional dead ends, the practical implications of those discoveries are staggering.

For example, mental hospitals, even at their very best, still disadvantage their patients by the stigma of having required the services of these institutions. Hospital records attach labels, accurate or otherwise, which often disrupt careers because they follow clients throughout their lives. A sad but necessary price? Some who say "No" would prefer to solve the problem by eliminating the services. This may be seductive as a cost-cutting measure, but it is potentially devastating for the patient. A transpersonal or human potentials approach to this problem would convert the hospital into an institute or school that could service people at all levels of health. As individuals learned to improve whatever skills they arrived with, diagnostic labels would give way to progress markers; the services would remain but the stigma would disappear. An entire community could use the institution; while one person worked through the infantile behaviors of a type of psychosis, another might try to improve a photographic memory or reduce blood pressure through meditation. Accomplishments at every level would be acknowledged and documented.

The transpersonal psychologist has shifted to this approach because of his basic belief that all people can choose to grow and, assisted properly, will succeed at it. In this way, science is refocused as a favored approach to improve our abilities and human potentials are continually redefined by the tools and techniques of the transpersonal movement.

In fact, the entire human potentials movement, because of its great variety of techniques, can focus on a multitude of interventions including psychodrama, sensitivity training and group encounter. Transpersonal psychology clearly is aimed at the balanced development of individual definition through integrating psychosocial disciplines and processes.

In the area of education, human potentials owe a considerable early debt to A.S. Neill, the headmaster of the Summerhill Free School whose concepts of learning stressed facilitation of a child's freedom of choice, emotional growth, empathy, self-motivation and positive world outlook. Neill demonstrated how schools can teach (for better or for worse) mental health and human potentials, as well as math, English and geography.

As with all branches of human studies (especially gerontology), we find that the earliest years contain the most promising potential for the entire lifespan. We also might note that the completion of compensatory education's first decade was marked by new visions of a child's potential. In the 1970s, education began offering to the students new roles by blurring the distinction between student and teacher. In recent years educational authorities have shown even more willingness to recognize individual differences in children, the teaching styles they respond to, and the favorable rate at which they learn.

Psychologist Tom Toy and I conducted a program to find out why tutored children learn twice as much as the untutored, and why the high school students who did the tutoring learned three times as much as their charges. We suggested setting up an educational cooperative in which every child had the opportunity to learn by teaching. Let me elaborate.

The striking achievements of tutors, even greater than those of their pupils, needed some thought and further exploration. In this study it seemed that identifying with the problems and the process of

Growing Younger

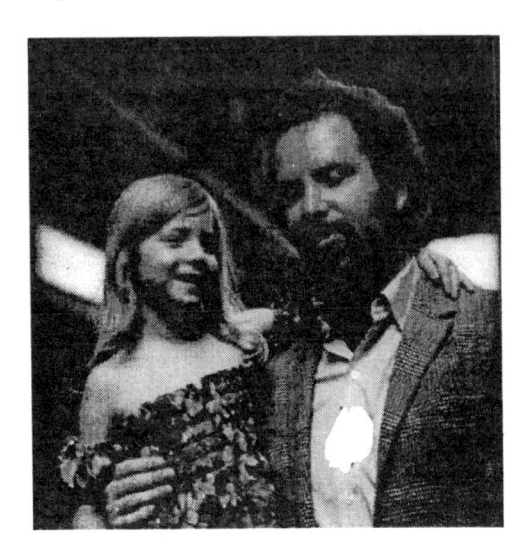

Loving children offer a magnificent trade: helping them grow older may keep you younger. Photos show Dr. Morgan with his daughters. *Top photo courtesy of Dr. Morgan. Below, photograph by David Gee.*

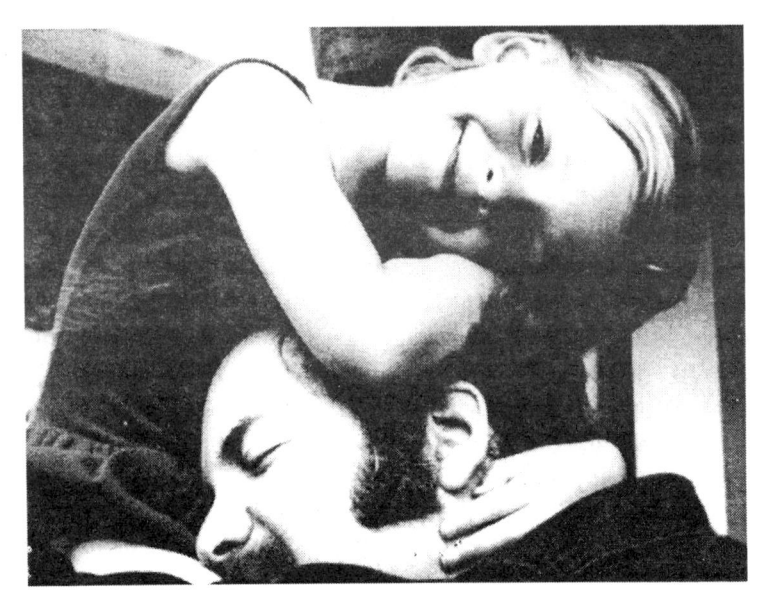

Looking Beyond Preconceptions

teaching others helped the tutors in their own classrooms. Yet, more seemed to be occurring than simply a role reversal of teacher-pupil identity; the tutor also had the opportunity to review material he had not seen in years and to master it fully. Without second chances like these, small deficits in reading or math can snowball over the years, making further education less rewarding with each succeeding year. This compensatory ploy of teaching content in order to *really* learn it is highly familiar to most university professors.

Whatever the reason, we found that teaching facilitated learning. The time our student tutor spent away from his study enhanced both his own education and that of his pupils.

One new approach to learning would be a total change in classroom atmosphere, expanding on the shared roles of student and teacher so that the undeclared war of mistrust between class and mentor could reach an honorable peace. To do this, teachers would have to acknowledge their responsibilities to all their students while at the same time acknowledging the students' potential ability to guide their own growth.

Tom and I proposed an educational system that would be a joint enterprise between children and adults. Responsibilities, roles and rewards would be shared. The unused pool of talented teaching manpower—the children themselves—would be funneled into the learning process. As much as half a child's time in school would be devoted to teaching and related duties (including administration or services). The students would teach children younger than themselves while learning from older children. The adult teachers would be the class organizers, the curriculum chiefs, the catalysts, and the professional consultants to this corporate enterprise. (They would even maintain an interest in keeping up on their subjects, including learning from their junior teachers.) For true sharing in such a system, rewards would be as relevant as roles and responsibilities. Therefore, one might use a graduated pay scale; one that would increase for all, based on the number of years in the school, with increments for additional duties or special achievements. In this system students would share everything of concern to their teachers—including a paycheck. I would guess that the drop-out rate and morale problems would be minimal in such a system. In fact, the huge manpower pool tapped, as well as the increased outside revenue (for holding more students in school longer) should make the higher salaries pay for themselves.

Growing Younger

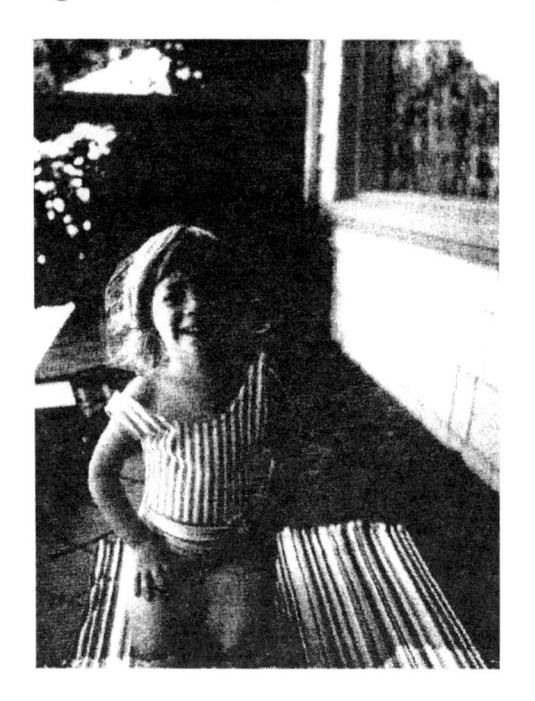

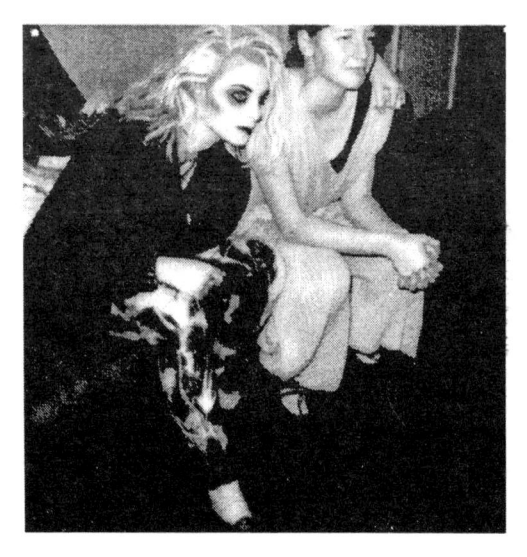

Looking Beyond Preconceptions

Naturally, teachers in such a system would have to be (or become) unusually secure, confident, intelligent and creative professionals. Since our children are often limited by the capacities of even the best teachers, they would surely benefit. It might be one of the few systems built around the needs of the child *and* the teacher, instead of one to the exclusion of the other.

Half of the waking hours of millions of teachers and children are spent in structured activities that seem devoid of personal meaning or fulfillment. The educational cooperative is a system that attempts to add meaning and purpose to education; something that seems more than a little needed these days.

Incidentally, the work done by Tom Toy and myself was combined with several other approaches and subsequently developed into what is called the Keller Plan or individualized (progress-at-your-own-rate-until-you've mastered-it) learning a system now often used in universities. Some day, perhaps, it will also become part of the pre-school and elementary system, where it is most needed.

How does all this apply to aging? You may remember that body temperature and metabolism can influence long-term survival if neurotic energy, stress and trauma are reduced. Therefore, effective personal growth also should help quite a bit. You will recall the potent roles played by auto-hypnosis and the self-fulfilling prophecy. Clearly, a good educational system can enhance a person's view of himself and make him better able to live a rewarding and meaningful life. That should help too. Beyond education, growth and psychotherapy, a personal focus on continued growth with specific transpersonal techniques also could affect aging.

Without rerunning the history of biofeedback, it can be pointed out that already it has been used effectively to reduce blood pressure and heart rate, which of course can influence human survival positively. Biofeedback is any method that can signal to individuals some degree of success in voluntarily changing aspects of their bodily processes that they ordinarily would not be able to measure. This signaling or feedback allows control over many body processes thought, no more than a decade ago, to be beyond cortical or deliberate voluntary control. Heart and temperature measures seem to be of the greatest interest to gerontologists. Immediate feedback allows them to observe a kind of instrumental conditioning to take place as

Growing Younger

subjects learn to do more with their bodies than they were able to do before. Biofeedback is a social phenomenon that should be taught to children as part of their regular school program. It reflects the increasing emphasis we place on mind and body as one unit. It is a very human adaptation of technology, allowing us to learn more about ourselves by controlling our mind-body functions. Biofeedback has been tried with aged volunteers to encourage faster brain wave responses and speed up reaction times; Cay Luce's SAGE project in Berkeley uses it as a growth technique for citizens over 80. How it affects the rate of aging still needs to be tested.

Effective mediation allows concentration on a single thought that could help the body to relax fully, if it could provide a more positive world view, greater resistance to stress, and increased personal energy. Is this then a rejuvenating process? To determine whether one method is better than another when measuring the effects of aging still remains to be tested. Transcendental meditation, for instance, is at once a philosophy, a business, a technique and a social movement. Research suggests that it can affect body age positively, over time, but replication is still needed to prove it.

Yoga in its many varieties is probably the most popular among the many exercise, breathing and energy-raising techniques. But actually *any* effective exercise regimen will offer some braking mechanism to the causes and effects of aging. Regular exercise also has a potent impact on the risk of coronaries. H.A. deVries, in his book *Vigor Regained,* found that men 60 to 90 years old responded well to two months of careful but vigorous exercise (calisthenics, jogging, etc.). They regained muscle tone and strength, their blood pressure dropped and their oxygen capacity was bolstered. DeVries recommends rhythmic exercise (e.g., fast walking) when the heart rate is at least 40% over resting (but not beyond 75%); he feels that much of what we consider aging is actually damage done by too much inactivity. Physical training can correct a full age-related range of morphological and motor fitness deterioration. Body age proof? Not yet, although early studies are encouraging. Already, some yoga and exercise classes have begun to use body age testing to measure individual client benefits. For some of us, the best human potentials exercise of all is to play with our children and adult partners.

Looking Beyond Preconceptions

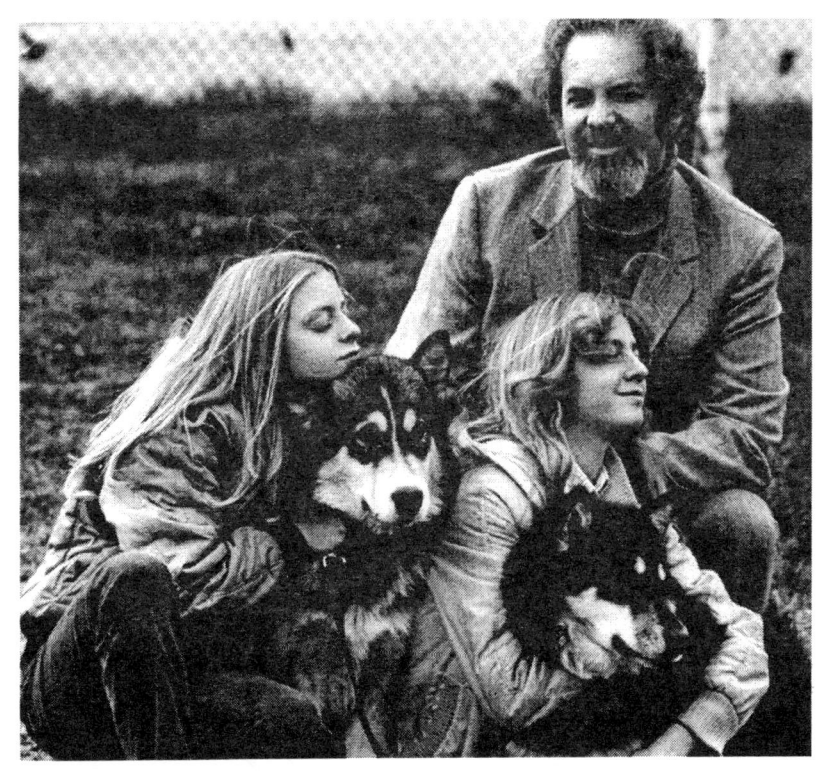

For some of us the best human potentials exercise of all is to play and relax with our children and adult partners. Above, author with Cinnamon and Angel-Kwan-Yin. *Photograph by Dwight Storring.*

In 1968. Duke University's John B. Rhine suggested that telepathy could be enhanced by hypnosis and other altered states of consciousness. Soviet scientists have already developed training programs for *psi* ability (E.S.P.) and even the cosmonauts used telepathy as an alternative signaling system when in orbit. This blend of biophysical technology and what was once considered an arena for mystics and frauds has revolutionized our thinking about the real world and our place in it. Peter Tomkins and Christopher Bird, in their book *The Secret Life of Plants* have helped in this regard. They maintained that wired-up plants demonstrated incredible sensitivity to humans under the right conditions—enough to shake a humanistic vegetarian. Parapsychology, including telepathy, is now considered a legitimate area for scientific inquiry, even by official division status in the American Association for the Advancement of Science. Soon we may find training programs in schools (neighborhood children already have had telepathy-based card-guessing games they routinely play with friends) and special therapy for those who lack minimum skills. Their deficiency, by the way, is called "Psi Missing," although it more often is a psi ability used against oneself. A person with psi missing might dig for gas and instead may find a buried outhouse. My own theory is that psi ability, particularly telepathy, may be a natural human skill that unless properly developed in infancy is lost to most of us in adulthood. Fortunately, the loss could be reversed. Yet at the present time, telepathy as an art is somewhat analagous to high-wire walking. Only a few can do it routinely and most of us not at all. One interesting exception: Eloise Shields of the Los Angeles County School noticed extraordinary telepathy skills in retarded children aged 5 to 21 (mean IQ 45). Her findings readily agree with the transpersonal bias that people at the bottom of one ability dimension can fit in at the top of another. Perhaps it is more than fitting in; rather, one ability compensates for the other. Clearly, we need more research in the field. How psi ability could affecting aging, I don't know; it remains to be tested.

What of the LeBoyer method of birth without violence—how might this revolutionize aging? My guess is, quite a lot. But the children so born are still a decade too young to test. A follow-up study by psychologist Danielle Rapoport on a sample of 120 children aged one to three, who were born by the LeBoyer method, revealed that they had a superior developmental quotient (six points above average) and virtually no mental health difficulties. They were alert, inventive and well co-ordinated, and 93% had never experienced difficulty in suckling or toilet training. All the children were born in a conventional working-class public clinic in Paris; therefore, their success was not due to the middle.. class benefits of extra money or an enriched environment. Rapoport thought the absence of difficulties in sleeping or feeding may have promoted the obviously above-average parent-child relationships observed. Clinics now practicing the LeBoyer method report a postnatal mortality decrease of 40% (12 per thousand from 20 per thousand). LeBoyer has already been on a speaking tour of North America and the method is suddenly as

Looking Beyond Preconceptions

sought after here as it is in France. In North America it is generally offered under the name Wholistic Childbirth (no pun intended, I think). A list of practitioners qualified to deliver babies in this may be obtained from IWC (Institute for Wholistic Childbirth), 1627 Tenth Avenue, San Francisco, California 94122. The list includes information for parents-to-be on communication, attention, the handling and massage of babies, and facilitating growth in the new relationship. Body age? Well, give it time.

At the other end of the age spectrum is SAGE (already mentioned), a holistic program for the growth and development of the over-SO generation.

Looking in new directions, how would multiple-marriage configurations affect aging? Would living according to the mores of a more psychologically sophisticated dream culture such as the Senoi in Malaya impact on our growth and youth? The renewed interest in life and self-responsibility is based on a background of genuine accomplishment: through relaxation training, biofeedback, hatha yoga, gestalt therapy, massage, meditation, tai chi, art and music therapy and instructive videotapes the person grows in an obvious self-chosen way. Enhanced abilities lead to a new view of one's own potential. SAGE even confronts death fears much in the same way that we attacked senility a decade ago. It is usually done with non-senile people in a preventive way. In short, a whole arsenal of transpersonal psychology is available and it seems to work.

And yet, a word of caution: too often, after one successful experience, healthy skeptics may become converts and missionaries. Keep your skepticism in order to balance an open mind. Explore each of these opportunities with caution and vision, and choose wisely before doing any missionary work. Not all friends are as open minded as you are; be sensitive to this and hold forth only when welcomed. Some people are deeply committed to not knowing what you or I could tell them. Probably the best transpersonal technique of all is to teach by example.

Growing Younger

~9~
Looking at
EACH OTHER
Work, Sex, Love and Purpose

DO WORK, SEX, LOVE and purpose all affect Our rate of aging? The conservative answer is yes—very much so.

Work
Satisfying work continued throughout life can lead to slowed aging and longer life. It was a common characteristic in the three long-lived cultures visited by Sula Benet and Alexander Leaf. The post-100 generation had meaningful tasks to perform and did them well. Similar findings come from decades of long.-term studies performed to date; one of them found that four out of every five 92-year-olds interviewed were working at least part time and many attributed their vigor to a refusal to take life easy.

On the other hand, forced retirement can be hazardous to our health. Certainly, we should retain the option to retire with continued income from an oppressive job. But meaningful, systematic, varied and paid activity should be available to adults of all ages. In many occupations (science, arts, agriculture) ability does not decrease or cease at age 65 and, in fact, those who continue to use it show significantly fewer signs of illness and a delay in accelerated aging. Rapid aging and death often come on the heels of retirement. This applies to whatever age a specific culture defines as its retirement age. Our culture sets one of the earliest retirement ages *(65)*. But in countries where manpower is limited, retirement comes much later. When jobs are scarce and seniority expensive, it is to the advantage of business and labor to retire personnel sooner (at perhaps

Growing Younger

less than half their lifespan potential), or so conventional wisdom has decreed in the past. The concept of forced retirement originated in Germany in the 1880s, when the custom of the employees of German insurance companies to retire at 65 was written into the entire country's social security system. When the United States established its social security system, it was modeled on that of Germany—Canada followed later. Soon the post-65 retirement years were defined as the years of "old age." The only people exempt from forced retirement were individuals who had their own businesses or those with independent spirits; only they had the freedom to sidestep the system and escape subsequent inactivity.

Is work defined as a salaried job, or can any regular, interesting mental or physical labor mean the same thing? Results suggest that while mental activity is probably the more potent of the two, physical activity is crucial to survival.

Like nearly all anti-aging aspects, regular exercise is more effective if begun early in life and continued throughout the entire lifespan. Although too little exercise is debilitating to the system, too much may be counter-productive. Intramural college athletes live longer than non-athletes, but major competitive athletes live briefer lives than non-athletes. More successful athletes probably absorb more stress and physical punishment. In other words, while enjoying regular exercise is conducive to greater survival, overly strenuous competition is not.

Whatever you contribute to society at age *64*, mentally and physically, cannot be without value a year later. If you continue to grow, there is no need to become useless. Fortunately, the over 65 generation has begun to be aware of this and now is sufficiently well organized economically and politically to do something about it. In the next five to ten years, look for real changes in our retirement process. We may be moving to a system in which it is normal to have three or four (20-year retirement) careers in a lifetime that will allow workers to collect a pension from. each job before moving on to the next.

Sex

H.L. Mencken defined puritanism as the haunting fear that someone, somewhere, may be happy. In these days of greater sexual freedom, it is still shocking to many that sensuality and sexuality are sought and enjoyed by the young and old as well as the middle-aged. Today junior is exposed to better sex education than ever before and can consult a wide variety of manuals. On the other hand, he is exposed to epidemic social diseases and sexploitation films. Grandma and Grandpa are being adequately counseled by many professionals that it is OK for them to continue their sex life. The truth is even stronger than that; a continued sex life, throughout the life span, seems to be a powerful anti-aging treatment.

At the Netherlands Cancer Institute it was discovered that old male rats lived significantly longer and in better health when young female rats were introduced into their cages. A team of Israeli scientists pursuing rat studies on the effects of celibacy found that the reproductive organs of unmated males were 35 to 40% smaller than those of mated males, with concurrent degeneration of the testes and coagulating glands, but that the atrophy of sex organs was reversible upon prolonged contact with females. It was also noted that unmated males averaged 72% more body fat. Whether this was solely due to lack of coital exercise or whether the body has its own fat-prone reaction to celibacy was not clear; what did become clear, however, was the fact that the fat was not advantageous to survival. Unmated rats averaged 578 days of life; mated ones 734 days—a 27% advantage. The mated rats were leaner, more resistant to disease and more vigorous, as well as possessing more fully-developed reproductive organs. When normally mated rats were prevented from mating. their disease resistance was lowered and their body fat increased substantially, although they were not eating any more. Mated rats also had 43% more testosterone.

But rats are not human beings, and body age measurement has been used to determine that people reporting an above average level of sexual activity were usually chronically happy—a trait linked to slowed aging.

People in Turkey who live past 90 typically maintain regular sex lives. Sex, therefore, may not only be the best exercise; it may also create a greater resistance to disease. Single men have twelve times greater chance of dying from tuberculosis than married men; single women are fifteen times more likely to die of heart disease. Average intercourse accounts for 200 calories; daily sex burns off 30 pounds a year of excess body fat—perhaps one of the more agreeable ways to lose weight.

In yet another rat study, arsenic was injected into the rodents to determine lethal thresholds. Mated males died at three times the dose at which celibate males succumbed; mated females had four times the resistance of their celibate sisters.

Shunamitism was a common practice throughout medieval Europe and in ancient Asian and middle-eastern cultures. The term is derived from Abishag, the Shunamite, a beautiful young woman who allegedly extended the life of King David of Israel in his old age, and subsequently extended the life of his son Solomon. Shunamitism was also a common practice in Northern India a thousand years ago and undoubtedly has arisen in many other cultures at different times. In medieval Europe. a common treatment for the pains of old age was for the male patients to sleep between two young girls, but the benefits probably extended to both sexes.

Sex differences have not yet been adequately explored in relation to aging. For example, even though every "rat" psychologist knows that male rats are less excitable than females, so far proof of this has always been confounded by the incontrovertible fact that both male and female rats (and humans) are the 50—50 genetic products of a male and female, just as male and female hormones, in varying proportion, can be found in each rat and every human regardless of sex. Further, the majority of rats and humans are raised in the presence of adults of both sexes. Perhaps we need a new approach to assess the genetic basis for behavioral differences between the sexes. Here is a hypothetical and fictitious study to test this theory:

> The first step is to sort laboratory rats by gender. Female couples are housed in individual cages in one room; male couples in a second room. Next, we apply the most familiar method for assessing genetic effects on behavior. Using a selective breeding procedure for at least ten generations, males are mated to males and females to females. Just as selective breeding has attempted to produce "intelligent" strains of rats, so we intend to produce "all male" and "all female" strains of rats as grist for serious behavioral as-

sessment. At present, sexually isolated, single-sex rat couples have been observed to be co-operative, even friendly, but the first litter is slow in coming!

I believe that celibacy can be hazardous to your health, although I do not expect such a statement to come from a Surgeon General of any country. In the interim, I have asked the Diagnostic and Statistical Manual people to at least list celibacy as a sexual deviation.

How much benefit stems from the act of intercourse alone and how much from emotional components? The question "is it sex or is it love?" is an over-simplified way of looking at the problem. Evidence seems to indicate that both as exercise and as emotional release, intercourse is in itself beneficial; further, hormonal and disease-resistant advantages seem likely.

Love

The heightened impact of that emotional state we term "love" may prove to be of great importance to the conquest of aging. In the eighteenth century, Benjamin Rush, a physician known as the father of American psychiatry, found that he had met only one person beyond the age of 80 who had never married. In modern times, insurance companies know that unmarrieds are at a much greater risk of early death than marrieds. An analysis of 3.5 million deaths proved that 55% of the deceased were widowed, single, separated or divorced. The death rate for both sexes (over age *55),* was twice as high for the single, separated or divorced as for the marrieds. Interestingly, widowed spouses had a lower death rate than divorced spouses. For example, death rates per 1,000 for those aged 65-74 were:

Men—married 42.3, widowed 72.5, divorced 96.7
Women—married 21.6, widowed 33.7, divorced 45.9.

This suggests that termination of a relationship by death is less traumatic than termination by voluntary decision or rejection. Studies also tell us that intact satisfying marriages are strong predictors of greater longevity. Modern techniques are available for assessing this factor, particularly in terms of the stress of required social readjustment when a relationship goes sour. Freud has told us that a

Growing Younger

measurement of normality is the ability to do well at love and work. Yet, psychoanalysis in this regard has not yet become a sufficiently pervasive part of our culture, especially of our early education.

Can we promote long life by strengthening the love aspects of human relationships? Should we begin young by setting up sexually-liberated "children's villages" like those reputedly common in southern India? Does the answer lie in polygamy, multiple marriages or communal living; or in greater self-understanding and maturity? Clearly, this is an area for much serious thought. There is no doubt that deep and meaningful relationships affect life itself.

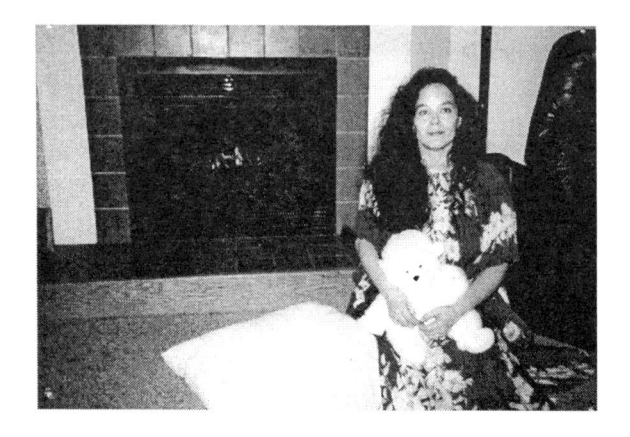

There are two sides to everything.

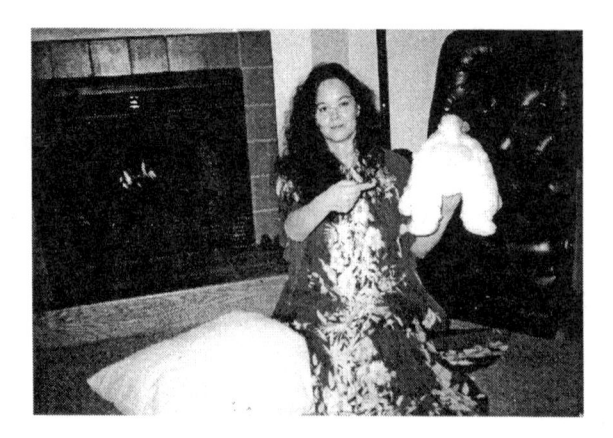

Purpose

Purpose is the explanation you give yourself for your continued existence. For some of us, work, sex or love may be a sufficient purpose for living. The Abkhasians, who work until they are well past 100, remain an active and respected part of their communities until death. Their culture seems to provide them with a strong enough reason to live on.

Mental activity through education and social programs may even be a more potent tool than physical activity in the retardation of aging. In a study done by psychologists Alice Dawson and Warren Baller at the University of Omaha, it was found that an 18-week oil painting course affected the longevity of the students, who were all over the age of 65. The 30 people who had enrolled in the course were twice as likely to be alive when followed up twelve years later than the 21 others who were used as a control group. The median age of the students at the time of the course was 70; all were retired. Twelve years later, only one-third of the art students had died, while two-thirds of the controls were no longer living; 65% of the surviving students were in good to excellent health while only 12% of the controls could be so rated. The 18 weeks of oil painting had been focused on developing creative expression as a means of relating to others. While most participants did not keep up their hobby, the initial experience nevertheless seemed to have helped them develop a post-retirement purpose for living and, perhaps, establish a social network of peers with a similar purpose. In Australia, psychologist and gerontologist Elsie Harwood uses "geriatric re-activation" to teach purposeful skills to retirees. She has been quite successful in forestalling both physical and mental deterioration through the 90s by using activities such as acting, language, music, dancing, swimming (life saving) and speech in the face of severe initial disabilities.

Professionals are most likely to maintain a high post-retirement purpose. Prominence and recognition are also good predictors: people over 45 who are listed in *Who's Who* are more likely to live longer than the general population.

The best time to develop individual purpose is in childhood, at the beginning of life. But when it comes to aging, our research suggests that no age group is too old to start. Post-retirement depression often begins with the question: "What am I living for?" It is initially

Growing Younger

stated negatively: "I have nothing to live for"; then dependently: "Tell me why I should bother to live"; and eventually, the question becomes part of the answer: "We live to learn why we are alive." By continually answering this question, our lives are made more interesting.

Here is a little story to illustrate that no age group is too old to develop purpose:

> In a small windowless room of a university, an administrator, four faculty members and a visiting dignitary hold an hour-long conference. The dignitary has the power to grant the school a lot of money. His first offering, however, is an involuntary burst of flatulence, so foul that the stench penetrates every corner of the room before the tell-tale thunderclap completes its reverberation.
>
> The administrator bursts into a broad smile and compliments the dignitary on his tie.
>
> The first faculty member, a full professor, breathes naturally, thinking "I've smelled worse."
>
> The second, an associate professor, breathes with some difficulty, but manages, eventually, by thinking about the foods that might have created the smell.
>
> The third, an assistant professor, holds his breath thinking, "Well, I'm leaving soon anyway."
>
> The fourth faculty member is a part-time instructor who retired the year before and feels totally comfortable with herself. She opens the door and, before stepping outside announces loud and clear, "Let me know when you're through farting around; my time is too valuable to waste."

Some Ideas on Work, Sex, Love and Purpose

Do changes (in any of these four dimensions) alter your rate of aging?

Are people who are satisfied with themselves different from those who are not, with regard to their rate of aging?

Why is life worth living? How satisfied are you with your answer? Can you increase your satisfaction?

~10~
Looking at
THE CLOCK
Time and Aging

THE PASSAGE OF time is not necessarily a linear, regular or easily measured process. Physicists and novelists from Einstein to Vonnegut have told us that time is also a place, with a variable geography. There are several psychological parallels to this concept, because even when we age at a normal rate, the experience of time can be altered.

In this chapter we will examine ways to increase our life span by living more fully in time, rather than by slowing our biological passage through it. There are anecdotes about those who came close to death and lived years of memories in seconds. We also have heard stories about people dying of a terminal illness, yet able to expand hours into centuries by the selective use of psychoactive drugs.

In 1948, Linn Cooper, a physician and hypnotist from Washington, D.C., published a study entitled "Time Distortion in Hypnosis"—time distortion being the process of experiencing much in short intervals, or little in long ones. In other words, a person properly hypnotized could experience an hour in 60 seconds of clock time. At that time, the phenomenon we now call "time acceleration" created a furor among psychologists and hypnotists. Did the subject really experience a minute of time for every second of clock time, or was the subject only hypnotized to think that this was so? Did the person actually undergo a biological acceleration or was it merely the experience of time that was affected? Could more be accomplished by accelerating time, and would this give us more time to think, or to solve mathematical or personal problems? Would our reflexes speed up or slow down proportionate to the distortion of time?

Growing Younger

Two years later, Dr. Cooper teamed up with the world-famous medical hypnotist, Milton Erickson. Together they defined time distortion as the marked difference between the seeming duration of a time interval and its actual duration as measured by the clock. They told of a boxer who was able to use time distortion to slow down (his experience of) his opponent to better place his punches. This is similar to baseball player Hank Aaron's description of how he saw baseballs move "in slow motion" when he was up to bat. We heard of the little boy who was hypnotized for dental work and saw a complete movie in the few minutes of drilling, and of the patient who spent one subjective hour working on his personal problems while devoting only 60 clock seconds to the task. Some people relived several hours of past experiences in just a few minutes of clocked therapy time. Hours of piano practice were experienced in minutes of hypnotized time. After Cooper and Erickson had investigated a number of case histories in time distortion, they concluded that "thought, under time distortion, while apparently proceeding at a normal rate from the subject's point of view, can take place with extreme rapidity relative to world time. Such thought may be superior, in certain aspects, to waking thought." Hypnosis was successfully used to alter the experience of time. Clearly this mid-century breakthrough offered some intriguing possibilities to time-conscious North Americans.

The history of the study of time distortion followed the history of hypnosis; over the decades it gained and lost respectability with the North American scientific and medical communities many times over.

Cooper had used the term "time distortion" exclusively for incidents in which hypnotized subjects had sped up experiential time (e.g., seeing a three-hour movie in ten clocked minutes). Then in 1958, Erickson published an article in which he distinguished incidents in which subjective time was slowed from those in which subjective time was accelerated. When subjective time was slowed, he called it "time expansion"—experiencing much in short intervals. But when subjective time was speeded up, it was termed "time condensation"—experiencing very little in long intervals. When you are "on the spot," so to speak, time expansion can be used to slow down the world to give you more time to think before acting. Time con-

Looking at the Clock

densation, on the other hand, can be used to speed up the (perceived) world—time spent standing in a long line, for example, could be made to pass very quickly. Perhaps a good analogy would be running a film at either slow- or fast-forward; a diver could take minutes, for instance, to reach the water surface, or a building could be completed in seconds, depending on how fast the film was run. In effect, both Cooper and Erickson helped their subjects alter the rate of the "filming" of their own life, as it occurred, or as it was rerun.

Philip Zimbardo, a noted author and social psychologist, is among those who use hypnosis to expand the present and abolish the future. He believes that our notion of time is the result of socialization and is used to regulate our behavior by forcing us to evaluate the present within the confines of the past and the future. Religion raises the specter of the past while at the same time promising better things to come. Art can impose a notion of timelessness on history. This notion enables us to live together, by transforming us from egocentered, impulsive creatures into social beings who can control the urge for gratification by subjugating the present, so that we can live by the lessons of the past and in anticipation of the future. In order to gauge the effects of time disortation, Zimbardo embarked on a study to see whether he could expand the present and diminish the restraints imposed by the past and the future. In this way he hoped to "liberate" his subjects, to make them more impulsive, irrational and chaotic—living for the moment.

Thirty undergraduate students (fifteen men and fifteen women) from Stanford University were chosen for the project. All checked out on a standard scale as potentially good hypnotic subjects. They underwent hypnotic training, directed toward teaching each one to perform self-hypnosis. Twelve members of the group received the hypnotic suggestion "to allow the present to expand and the past and future to become distanced and insignificant." The other eighteen were given a variety of instructions, some relating to time-distortion recorded on tape; other members were told to imagine how a hypnotized subject would respond and then act as if they were hypnotized. Some were given time-distortion instructions without hypnosis and some were left to experience time normally.

All the volunteers were asked to perform three tasks: first, they had to write stories about two pictures—one before and one after

Growing Younger

time distortion. Next, they had to listen to a humorous tape recording and write down their reactions. Last, they were each given a two-pound blob of clay and told they had five minutes to make something out of it.

What happened?

Hypnotized—Normal Time

The young lady is happy, looking at cows on the hill, she is peaceful. The old lady is

---
Hypnotized—Expanded Present

I am, but looking. They are looking for nothing, no one but being warm. They are in the sun feeling nothing but glaze. It is very very very quiet. It is very light. It is just Hum day being + rose

Both pictures chosen for the first task hinted at time themes. One showed an old woman and a young man, the other a farmer planting crops while a pregnant woman looked on. The hypnotized volunteers used more present-tense verbs in writing about the photographs and made fewer references to the future. The group simulating a hypnotic response outdid everyone else, using even more present-tense verbs and far fewer references to both past and future. Ob-

Looking at the Clock

serve the difference in handwriting in the sample on the preceding page, written by the same person before and after time expansion.

Everyone then listened to a five-minute pirated tape recording of an abortive radio commercial for an old movie *(The Caddie)*. The comedy team in the ad committed several blunders and lapsed into a verbal war by trading curses, criticisms and taunts. In doing so, their language grew more and more obscene. As the group listened to the tape, the judges recorded their reactions from behind a one-way mirror.

The hypnotized subjects laughed three times as often as any of the other volunteers. They were also the only ones to reflect the language used on the tape in their written answers. After the running of the ad, everyone had to fill out a questionnaire.

A typical view of the kind of unusual reaction generated by playing with time in this way became evident in the following report, written by a hypnotic subject one minute after hearing the tape recording.

> I don't remember much about it now—all I remember is that it was funny and that I'd seen the movie the men were talking about. But actually I don't really care too much about the tape at all right now. I hate writing this. So I'm stopping. Right now. I feel like laughing. But I'd better stop writing this first. Right now.

When the volunteers were ready to perform the third task (to make an object or a shape of out of clay in five minutes), Zimbardo expected that the group with an expanded sense of the present would be less likely to plan ahead and would end up with nothing distinguishable at the end of the allotted time. But the time proved too short for most of these subjects to complete any objects at all, and when they were told to finish up they hurriedly slapped something together.

Interestingly, the expanded-present subjects continued to play with the clay for four more minutes after having been told to stop. The normal-time volunteers finished before the original time had expired. Two-thirds of the hypnotic group showed no concern with being dirty or having their hands covered with clay. They also

Growing Younger

seemed to enjoy handling the clay more than the others. Almost all the other subjects cleaned up as soon as they had finished their work.

Here are the comments of the hypnotic subjects:

Felt like I was working in the dirt, like the farmer in the picture felt the soil under my fingernails, drying out and becoming like shaving talc.

The thing I like most about working with the clay is getting my hands dirty... all the clay I've got all over my hands now.

The thing I like least about working with the clay is the fact that it stuck to my hands and now I am a clayman.

My hands dirty afterwards, but that's O.K.

The clay was very soft and moist; it felt nice to dig my fingers into it. When I was working with it, the shape just kind of happened. There was very little effort involved. It just kind of worked itself out.

The subject who really enjoyed working with the clay was still very much in tune with the immediate present when she wrote:

I didn't want to stop. But now I don't care because I'm writing this. I've got clay on my hands. Now I'll move to question #1.
I remember feeling very, very, good. But that was clay and now this is pencil and paper. It's amazing how a pencil can make marks on a paper that other people can read and understand.... I can't really think about working with the clay. These questions interrupt my thought process. That makes me angry. But I don't care because it's all fantastically amazing. I can hear the blood in my ears.. .. Now I wonder why that is. No more room. Back in the folder.

Those who were quite distressed by the mess wrote:

Looking at the Clock

My hands are caked with clay, and I got some on my shirt.
It's a drag for my hands to feel like this.
I've got all this goddamn clay on my hands.
It got my hands dirty as hell.
It got clay under my fingernails and that's probably the most uncomfortable feeling I've had in 2 days.
It leaves your hands filthy.

In summing up his experiment, Zimbardo concluded that verbal instructions have a profound effect on the behavior of hypnotized subjects. "Their language changed toward more frequent use of present tense verbs, and more references to present events. They were more likely to laugh aloud at funny events and to continue to be preoccupied in a sensory experience. They were less concerned with their appearance and had more difficulty answering questions pertaining to memories of their reactions on prior experimental tasks."

Zimbardo suggests two very promising applications for this type of technique that could affect our aging. Senility is generally characterized by amnesia of recent events and a clear memory of past happenings. It could be that senile people, feeling a sense of hopelessness about both the present and the future, may be living in an expanded past. As an example, Zimbardo cites the case of the 68-year-old institutionalized patient who wished his face were a shirt he could launder, pack in a drawer and then take out fresh and unchanged whenever he needed it. "Perhaps," Zimbardo theorizes, "the aged put their memories in a drawer to be preserved against time." Do they not tell and retell stories about the past, tinging them with new significance and tender nostalgia? It seems that the present is uncomfortable and the future unthinkable. Through hypnosis and other techniques, people could attain longevity by expanding their sense of the present and the future.

Such time distortion also could be used in conjunction with hypnotically-induced age regression, to retrieve past events and overcome their negative effects. Zimbardo calls it "reweaving the past from the fabric of the present." It could smooth out the rough spots raised by statements such as "if only I'd known then what I know now."

The potency of a technique to influence not only time perspective but also self-image and inhibitions becomes evident in the spon-

Growing Younger

taneous reaction of a female volunteer who was concerned about being overweight. While in an expanded-present 1 state, she wrote:

> I'm melted, I am so thin, I cover practically everything. In fact, I am sort of falling into everything because lam so thin, and I can hear all the little things vibrating, and I can taste all the different things, like wood and the carpet, and the floor and the chairs, I really can't see any more, though, I mean it's all different colors, but it's so big you can hardly see it, everything is very confusing, but I've just sort of melted into every- -thing.... I'm unresponsible! ... I'm everything! I can keep going.... I'm not a thing anymore, I'm everything so I can't do anything. There's nobody there, nobody who says to me, 'Hey, Everything, you have to do this!'

The results obtained from Zimbardo's work therefore confirm that hypnotized time distortion exists above and beyond compliance, request or fraud. On the other hand, not every hypnotist can do it; nor is every subject equally capable.

We can speculate that if time acceleration can be used in conjunction with auto-hypnosis to control aging, the benefits would be great. With time distortions on demand, we could choose to speed up or slow down time as it suits our needs. Perhaps we could choose to accelerate or slow our physical speed (simple and complex reaction time, for example) as required, just as Elkind's study suggests that we can use hypnosis to slow the aging process itself. Such skills would and should be generally available to the public. I can even imagine a forward-thinking school adding them to its curriculum, especially at the primary level.

Do we need to be hypnotized or to be hypnotists in order to make better use of our time, to accelerate it if we choose? No, there is another way called temporal conditioning—learning to synchronize ourselves with intervals of time.

Do you know people who can automatically wake up at exactly the time they chose the night before? Or someone who can set an internal "alarm clock," perhaps using external clues (sunrise, birds, traffic, bladder, etc.)? Even in isolation you too can learn to synchro-

Looking at the Clock

nize with nearly any time interval. Russian scientists believe this can be accomplished by setting up a rhythm in the brain to alternately stimulate and inhibit electrochemical reactions.

In my own research, I devised a very basic technique to train the time sense. I seated my subjects in a dark, isolated room, lit with a light bulb that was geared to flash briefly at regular intervals. I asked them to say "NOW" when they felt the light was about to flash. The purpose of the game was to predict as closely as possible when the light would flash and to say "NOW" before it occurred. Everyone had fifteen tries, and the entire group became better at it as time went by. The most effective way to be right every time was *not* to count the minutes or the seconds, but to relax, because the body would tense just before a flash was due. The same experiment had been attempted both in the United States and in the USSR. Interestingly, American subjects succeeded at short intervals—up to 60 seconds, while the Russians required longer intervals—not less than 30 minutes in most cases.

My own work demonstrated that temporal conditioning was possible at both short and long intervals with a difficult period in between. But what was most relevant was an accident that occurred while the experiment was in progress. The volunteers needed for the long-interval studies were paid for a 16-hour day. They showed up expecting a series of experiments, not realizing that the entire 16 hours would be spent in a single study. As they entered the lab they noticed food and drink on the table and a urinal in the corner of the room... signs of a long stay. However, when they were told to say "NOW" just before the light flash, they didn't expect more than a minute or two between flashes. In fact, the intervals were 60 minutes, a full hour, fifteen times in a row. After the study it became clear that all the volunteers had underestimated not only the length of the intervals but also how long they had been in the lab. Sixty minutes was perceived to be five minutes, for example. One man was so convinced that he had been in the room for only one hour (rather than 16 hours) that he didn't use the urinal or eat any food during the entire time. This, of course, is a classic time-distortion technique in which the time rate is off by a constant factor. (For example, the hypnotist might say that each metronome click signifies the passage of one minute when in fact it signifies the passage of a second.)

Growing Younger

Weeks after the close of the study, one volunteer returned to me complaining that since his participation, time seemed to be flying by. "I get in a long line at the bank," he told me, "and before I can get out my checkbook the teller is there, waiting for me. People seem to be whizzing by me." To his wife and friends he appeared slow. He would no sooner sit down than they would point out that an hour had passed. In short, his time rate (experiential) had been accelerated or condensed and he did not like it.

I put him back in the room and applied "extinction" techniques by gradually synchronizing him with shorter and shorter time periods until we reached 60 seconds. He came back a second day and we did fifteen trials at 60-second intervals. After that, his time rate was normal again and remained that way.

When does time naturally accelerate for you? How might this affect measured aging? We can extend our active life to make better use of the time we have. You may wish to try some of these techniques to see if they can work for you.

Looking at the Clock

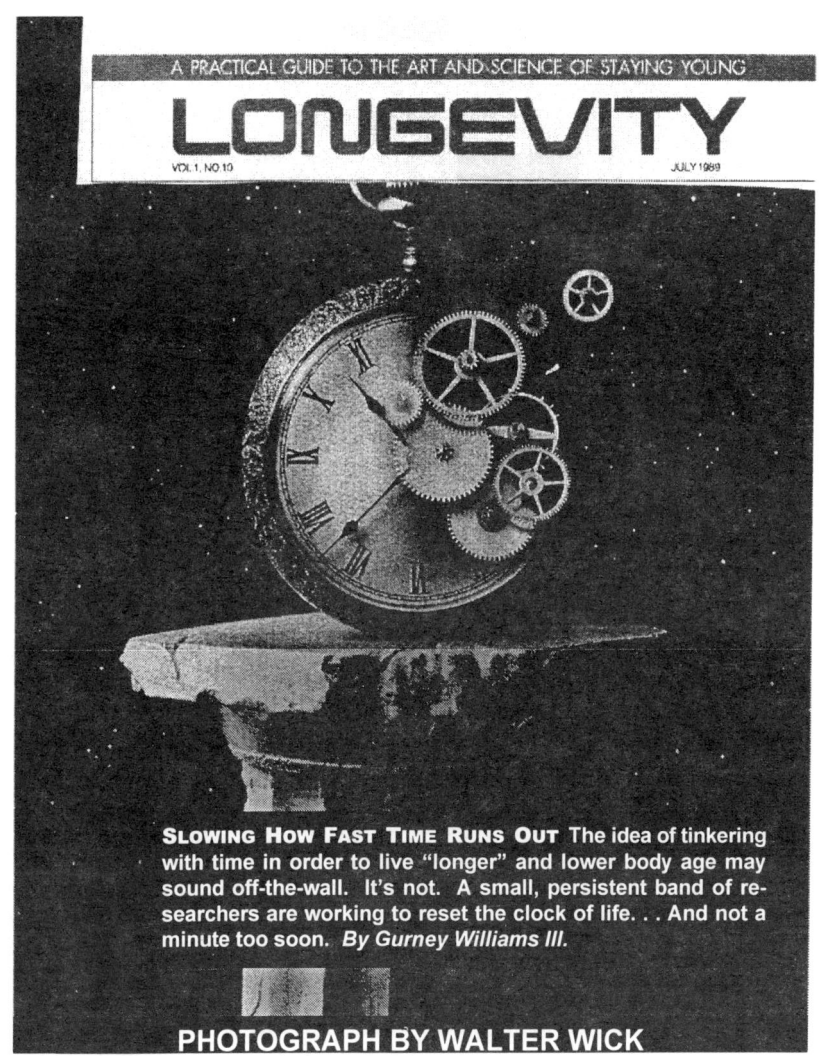

LONGEVITY
VOL. 1, NO. 10   JULY 1989

A PRACTICAL GUIDE TO THE ART AND SCIENCE OF STAYING YOUNG

SLOWING HOW FAST TIME RUNS OUT The idea of tinkering with time in order to live "longer" and lower body age may sound off-the-wall. It's not. A small, persistent band of researchers are working to reset the clock of life... And not a minute too soon. *By Gurney Williams III.*

PHOTOGRAPH BY WALTER WICK

SLOWING HOW FAST TIME RUNS OUT
BY GURNEY WILLIAMS III

Time flew, and it wasn't any fun. Charlie, 18, would stand in a long line at the bank and, it seemed, barely have a moment to pull out his checkbook before the teller yelled "Next!" at him. He would sit down for a chat with his wife and no sooner start talking before she would tell him an hour had passed. It seemed as though his life was skittering by in fast motion, like a Keystone Kops comedy. If Charlie lived to be 150, he would have felt shortchanged on time. Robert F. Morgan, Ph.D., then a graduate student at Michigan State University, took the blame. He knew immediately when Charlie—not his real name—came back to see him a week later that his experiment with time had gone too far. By manipulating a simple laboratory situation, Morgan had created a man who was living at fast-forward speed. Charlie was a student volunteer in a time-conditioning experiment Morgan was running at Michigan State. When he began, Morgan had no idea that it would so radically reset anyone's body clock. His goal had been simply to see whether people could improve their ability to guess how much time had passed between two events.

The experiment wasn't complicated. Charlie sat in a room bathed in dim red light. There were few comforts: chicken, lemonade, a glass urinal. The focus of the room was a 100-watt frosted light bulb a foot and a half in front of Charlie. It blinked on briefly, once an hour, for 16 hours. Charlie's only task was to guess when the light would go on and to say "Now!" just before the expected flash. No one told him how much time would pass between blinks. He had no idea how long the experiment would last.

In a separate room, Morgan monitored the experiment. Subjects wore two small electrically sensitive rings on their fingers to register the production of sweat, a sign of arousal or excitement. It was clear to Morgan as he watched the continuous readouts that his subjects felt a physiological twinge of anticipation just before they said "Now!" The signal that turned on the sweat, he concluded, came from some kind of mental clock.

In the course of 16 hours, the "clock" became more and more accurate in anticipating the next flash. After the first few hours, guesses frequently came within seconds of the light. But paradoxically, at the end of the 16-hour experiment Charlie and other subjects emerged bleary-eyed from the red room without any idea of what time it was.

Charlie told Morgan that he thought the whole session had taken just an hour, with the light blinking every four minutes. That's why he never ate any chicken or used the urinal, he explained: There just hadn't been time. He returned to daily life as a man running at 33 revolutions per minute (rpm) in a 78-rpm world. Acutely uncomfortable, he soon returned to Morgan for help.

To "reset" Charlie, Morgan put him back into the red-glowing room, told him again to try to anticipate when the light would go on and gradually shortened the period between flashes until the frosted bulb was blinking once every 60 seconds. It worked. Charlie's perception of time returned to normal. There was even a small payoff for his pain: Like most of the other subjects in Morgan's research, he stopped needing an alarm clock. His sense of time became acute enough to bounce him out of bed when he had to wake up.

Now a psychologist at the Pacific Graduate School of Psychology in San Francisco, Morgan is one of a mere handful of researchers exploring the passage of time. Their work helps explain why some car-accident victims review their whole lives in the split second before a crash. It's part of a primitive survival mechanism, according to David Cheek, M. D., a California obstetrician and a widely recognized expert on hypnotic states. "It's very important for animals to have instant replay of what permitted them to get out of trouble before, Cheek says. In humans the sudden deceleration of time as they hurtle toward collision allows for evasion or escape.

Perhaps most important, researchers have learned that no one needs to be a prisoner of time. Using autohypnotic techniques, there are ways to change our perceptions of how we're aging. Some therapists today are helping people travel in time—not only backward to retrieve the memories of youth but also forward to tap the wisdom of old age. Morgan's basic message: Time is largely subjective, every person's province to be conquered and controlled.

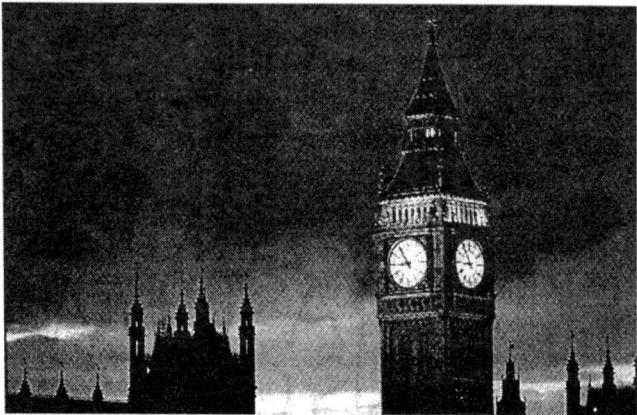

TIME-ZONE DEFENSE

Sometimes navigating between past, present and future takes the skills of a detective, psychologist Robert Morgan says. In one of his most memorable cases, a woman in her late 30s went to him for therapy because she suffered continual stomachaches. A series of gastrointestinal tests had turned up no obvious medical problems.

Her life story wasn't remarkable. She had moved from London to California 17 years before Morgan saw her, and she returned to London for occasional visits. She was married.

"How do you spend your day?" Morgan asked her. She said she drank a six-pack of Pepsi in the morning and smoked two packs of cigarettes by 2 p.m. Many therapists and physicians might have stopped there, having pinpointed a potential danger to her health. Sensitive to time, Morgan pressed on. "When do you eat?" he asked her. She said that at 2 p.m. she ate the first meal of the day. She felt hungry again at about 10 p.m. but fasted until well after midnight, when she ate a snack.

Morgan scribbled some time-zone calculations that led him to the root of her problems.

"You're living on London time," he told her, "and it isn't jet lag." Pepsi in the morning, California time, took the place of the tea Londoners were sipping at the same time. Her 2 p.m. meal coincided with a late dinner in London. The hunger pangs at 10 p.m. marked the time for breakfast in Hyde Park. But, like many Londoners, she skipped breakfast and ate only a light lunch—at three in the morning on the West Coast of the United States.

She had chosen to "live" in a comforting time zone, Morgan reports, far from the husband, whom—she soon acknowledged—she disliked and subsequently divorced. Then she automatically switched her body clock to local time.

Looking at the Clock

HOW LONG IS A MOMENT?

All of us experience time distortion, Morgan says. Classic childhood summers can seem to last forever, while the great getaway vacation often seems gone in an instant. 'The older we get," says Morgan, "the more time seems to speed' by." By contrast, some researchers speculate, everything seems sluggish to a newborn. The late anthropologist Margaret Mead once pointed out that the one-day-old child who has been wearing a wet diaper for half a day has been wet half his life. At any age, pain or frustration decelerates time an takes us back to that infantile sense that life is a river of molasses. Heavy traffic slows clocks. Bank lines seem to wind forever.

Animal studies reveal that at least some of our time perception is hardwired at birth. Different animals have divergent perceptions of how fast or slowly the world turns. The studies show that each species has a moment, the smallest

Perceivable time fragment. For humans the moment is one eighteenth of a second. If a reed vibrates more rapidly than that, you hear the vibration as a single tone. Eighteen taps applied to human skin in one second feel like a continuous touch. And 18 pictures projected per second on a screen look like one picture; our moment makes movies possible.

For the fighting fish, a freshwater animal that survives by catching fast-moving prey, research shows that the moment is one fiftieth of a second. To such a fish our movies would look choppy, and human swimmers would seem to

Move in slow motion. A snail moment, though, is only a third to a quarter of a second. Meandering brooks probably seem like white-water rapids to snails.

Although humans share a single moment, we differ in our personal time perspectives, according to Philip G. Zimbardo, a psychology professor at Stanford University. The perspective or "time zone," you're in, Zimbardo speculates, may reveal something about your health and potential longevity.

Growing Younger

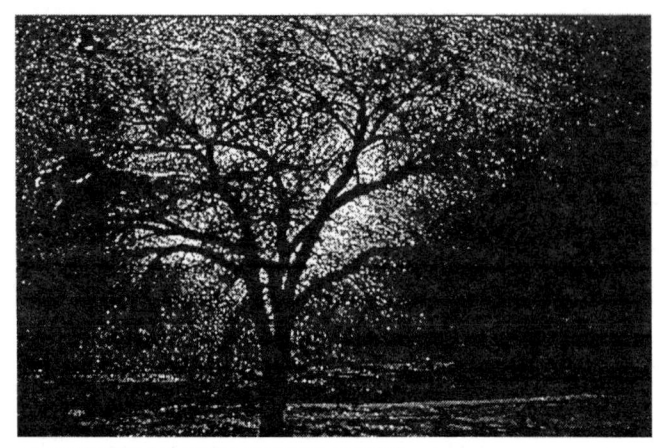

REWINDING THE BRAIN STEM
Recently I asked Sidney Rosen, M.D., a New York City Psychiatrist, to teach me how to distort my sense of the passage of time while under hypnosis. Here are portions of a transcript from a recent session. Rosen is speaking. I am awake at the start.
 "What we're going to do is get you to focus your attention on one thing. . . .It could be a thought you focus on, or it could be a word or a sound, a sensation. . . .
 "You can go into as deep a trance as you want, simply by focusing attention on whatever phenomenon interests you. . . .Your curiosity will guide you and lead you more and more into your trance.
 "Your breathing has become slower, your muscle tone has become more relaxed. . . .You can have a dream or see a movie right now. Your dream is just about ready to start, isn't it? Now. . . .[Twenty seconds pass.] is the dream all finished?
 "I'm going to count backward slowly from 20 to 1. I'd like you to come out of your trance one twentieth with every number that I count toward one, so by the count of one your eyes are open. You feel relaxed, rested, refreshed, wider and wider awake. . . ."
 He counted me out of the trance. When he told me to dream, I had climbed a tree self-consciously. It was a birch with scratchy white bark. I thought of Robert Frost's poem "Birches." At the top I looked around and saw dark skies and sensed the penetrating eyes of Sidney Rosen. The events in the dream seemed to take about a minute to unfold—but Rosen assured me that practice would help me "stretch" my experience of elapsed time in a hypnotic state. A *paradox*, I thought: *It takes time to get more time.*

HAZARDOUS TIME ZONES

Zimbardo and Alexander Gonzalez, chairman of the psychology department at California State University, Fresno, discovered seven such zones while studying over 12,000 responses to a national magazine reader survey. One zone, for example, is occupied by "Present, Fatalistic" people likely to say: "If things don't get done on time, I don't worry about it." Denizens of the "Present, Hedonistic" time zone believe that "getting together with friends to party is one of life's important pleasures" and say, 1 do things impulsively, making decisions on the spur of the moment." By contrast, future-oriented people—who occupy any of four distinct "Future" zones—are likely to map out their day every morning, take responsibility for deadlines and buy life insurance. The last of the time zones, the "Time Press" zone, is the realm of people inordinately preoccupied with punctuality and maintaining a tight schedule.

Zimbardo is currently mapping out the health-maintenance habits of people with different time perspectives. His suspicion: Life in some of the time zones may be hazardous to your health.

"Present, Hedonistic people are most prone to addictions," Zimbardo says, "things that feel good regardless of their long-term consequences. So I expect you get a high percentage of mortality among them because they get addicted to drugs, food, cigarettes." They are also less likely to carry out simple health-maintenance duties, such as setting up routine medical checkups. Beyond disco dancing, they tend to sit out strenuous exercise. Zimbardo lacks sufficient data to make similar predictions about Present, Fatalistic people, but chances are that their tendency to see life as something beyond their control puts them in at least as much jeopardy as their hedonistic counterparts.

People of the various Future zones are more likely to watch Their diets; exercise wisely and get the medical support they need.

Growing Younger

Zimbardo doesn't see much hope of transporting Present zone people into a healthier time zone. But Zimbardo and other researchers say that people in all chronological zones can change their *perceptions* of the passage of time. They point to the classic work done some 40 years ago by Milton H. Erickson, M.D., and Linn F. Cooper MID., who used hypnosis to create the human equivalent of the fighting fish—people who can, in effect, live "longer" by experiencing the passage of time more slowly.

PUTTING THE CLOCK ON HOLD

Erickson and Cooper called one of' their prize subjects 'E." Under hypnosis E. was 'told to imagine herself doing a repetitive task.' She used to have a job packing cookies, she said. Erickson told her to picture herself counting the cookies as she packaged them. After a set time, he told her to stop and describe everything that she had imagined herself doing.

She had been in a basement, she said, putting cookies into sacks. She counted out loud for Erickson to show how fast she had been working: one cookie per second. She had done it for 23 minutes, she said, time enough to pack about 1,400 cookies.

But there had been distractions. She had had a sneezing fit. The phone had rung for almost half the time she had been working. She let it ring and kept her count. By the end of the work session, she had packed 1,003 cookies.

"Was it real?" Erickson asked E. of her hypnotic dream.

"Yes," she said. Erickson had kept careful track of how much clock time had elapsed. E.'s 23 minutes had actually taken ten seconds.

Starting at the fifth second, Erickson had sounded a single note on a pitch pipe. E. said the phone had begun to ring as she was packing the four-hundred-ninety-eighth cookie, almost exactly halfway through her work.

Psychologists today who know Erickson's work are using

trances as a means of "stretching" time. Jeffrey Zeig, Ph.D., director of the Milton H. Erickson Foundation in Phoenix, follows Erickson's lead by punctuating his work as a therapist with personal mental forays into altered states where time seems to slow down.

SLOWING TIME TO LIVE LONGER MAY SEEM NUTS. IT'S NOT.

I set my mind on an idea, like *creativity* or *comfort,"* he says. Then he opens himself up to spontaneous images from his unconscious mind. His noonday trances last no more than 10 or 15 minutes each.,

Zeig says each of his trance states "seems pretty long," although he has never measured the dream events in his trances the way Erickson did to record the time expansion. "It's not a panacea," he cautions. "I'm still tired at the end of work." But the time distortion does help him attain a simple goal shared by most people: "I want to make five minutes of rest seem as long, as possible," he says.

A BRAKE ON AGING

Hypnotic time manipulation may offer more than relaxation. Although the evidence is sketchy, some therapists say hypnotic suggestion can directly slow the aging process or at least help in the treatment of physical and mental disorders. When Leonard Elkind, PhD,, a clinical psychologist in private practice in North San Diego, was a doctoral candidate in the early Seventies, he tested the anti-aging potential of hypnotic suggestion. Nineteen women took part in his experiment. Some were told: "Your body can become younger." All were given an examination called the AGE test, designed to assess how their bodies were aging. The 15-minute test, developed by Robert Morgan, measures hearing level at high frequency, the ability to read print close to the eyes and systolic, blood pressure, then generates a numerical "age" score that often differs from a subjects chronological age. Elkind's subjects, ages 39 to 56, had "body age" scores that ranged from 23 to 66.

Nine of the women were then hypnotized. "The body is a self-repairing organism," they were told while in their trance states. "Through hypnosis your body can become younger; not like a child but like a healthy, vigorous adult. . . .Let yourself feel younger. Feel the vigor and health that is yours. . . ." The remaining ten women served as controls.

Three weeks after the hypnotic session the whole group retook the AGE test. The members of the control group showed modest changes in body age. No subject's score differed more than four points from her first score, and some of them tested "older." But every member of the hypnotized group enjoyed a *drop* in body age, from three to 18 years. The median drop was 11 years.

In a related experiment cited by Morgan, a 59-year-old Canadian woman named Marg [sic] Meston, who had volunteered for a television demonstration, registered a body age score of 61 when first tested. Two months later, after posthypnotic suggestion, her body age had dropped to 40.

Elkind has not performed follow-up studies on his 19 subjects, nor have many investigators pursued this avenue of longevity research. The prospect of embarking on a longitudinal study in which the most salient data—dates of death—are, many decades away may be inherently daunting. Nonetheless, time distortion has become a mainstay of Elkind's work as a therapist. For many patients he prescribes what he calls a "time wedge." He tells patients to envision a place that's special to them. It may be a vacation retreat or a mountaintop with unlimited vistas. "Then at some point I'll remind them that in hypnosis, all time is *now* and that they have all the time they need for productive dreams." Patients wake up from these . five-minute trances feeling as though they've been "gone" for an hour—almost doubling their therapy time. Most important, says Elkind, patients in a time wedge may gain more freedom of choice.

"I call it a time Wedge because people sometimes find themselves in points in their lives when they see everything as black or white, either-or. The time wedge disrupts this either-or proposition." In a time-wedge trance, Elkind says, his patients have the extra time they need to consider new options for their lives.

He cites the case of a woman once tortured by a phobia about leaving her house and driving a long way to work on a California freeway. In hypnosis she has since learned to see the trip differently, helped by Elkind's suggestions that the frightening quantum leap from home to office is really just a connected series of short trips between freeway exits. The trance state gave her time to rehearse the journey in her mind until it wasn't alarming anymore. As a result, she has virtually stopped taking tranquilizers.

Using similar time wedges, therapists such as Jeffrey Zeig have helped women in childbirth stretch out periods of comfort between contractions. And by making the contractions themselves seem shorter, time-distortion techniques have reduced the demand for palliative drugs, making the birth process safer for mother and child.

FUTURE TENSE

Techniques that alter time perception offer fundamental gifts of longevity, Morgan says: a bonus of good time in your life. But you can also learn to live better in the present by mentally traveling to other times—most intriguingly, the future.

A 37-year-old Colorado woman was ambivalent about a divorce. Morgan hypnotized her, then told her to visualize her own face at age 57—two decades later—and listen to advice from herself. "She made contact," Morgan says, "and saw herself very dearly, but it was a tense encounter. It wasn't that she disliked her future face. The problem was like a broken TV: She saw a picture with no sound."

Explaining the uneasy silence, Morgan told her, "You

don't want to hear what you're going to say." In several subsequent sessions he taught the woman that she was just as free to ignore advice from her future self as from anyone else. With that reassurance, she began to hear her own voice, warning her against staying with her husband. She later acknowledged that she had been afraid that the figure in her future would tell her to avoid divorce at all costs—counseling that her mother might have given her.

"The permission to get the divorce wasn't just advice from a mother or wise person," Morgan says. It came from someone in her future who could reassure her—better than anyone else—that things were going to work out.

Whether the goal is resetting one's biological time clock, lowering body age, gaining an hour's worth of rest in a five-minute trance, using a time wedge to sort out tough choices—or even asking advice from an older and wiser version of oneself—the common message of time-oriented therapists and physicians is that you can use your mind to put time to work for you. The payoff may even be a longer life span, and if not that, then at least the *experience* of a longer life, with greater well-being. That, in the end, is arguably what longevity is all about.

Gurney Williams III is a writer and a lecturer on science, health and the future. He is also the **former editor of Omni.**

~11~
Looking at
MISTAKES
Iatrogenic Hazards
and Aging

IATROGENIC MEDICINE is the study of those diseases caused by the practitioner. When the treatment is worse than the actual illness, the effects generated by the curing agent become "iatrogenic." Unfavorable side effects can be due to drugs, surgery or therapy. So when you accidentally overhear your doctor say to his nurse, "Better get this patient back to surgery fast. We've discovered an iatrogenic problem," beware! He may well mean that a sponge has been left in your abdomen during your appendectomy.

The study of iatrogenic pathology is becoming more widespread as the focus shifts from the supplier to the consumer. Even medical patients are growing more aware of their right to know the consequences of a particular treatment. Informed consent and access to one's own files are part of this process; more fundamental and revolutionary would be the recognized legal right of any patient to independent before-and-after evaluation for any treatment received. Not only would this put the spotlight on iatrogenic "oopses," it also would identify techniques that work, and recognize effective practitioners. The right to know the truth is the prize of the past quarter-century, perhaps the long-sought prize of the scientific method itself.

Several years ago, I proposed that the *Diagnostic and Statistical Manual of Mental Disorders* published by the American Psychiatric Association add a new category entitled "iatrogenic disorders"—those caused by medical treatment and/or hospitalization. Chief among these would be:
- Institutionalization

Growing Younger

- Brain damage due to electroshock treatment
- Drug overdose and/or side effects
- Inadequate discharge planning
- Addiction to treatment (medical dependency) including prescription drugs.

The American Psychiatric Association didn't reply, but medical colleagues have pointed out that, while honest and scientific, such a diagnosis would instantly invite malpractice litigation!

How does this apply to longevity? In this context, I wish to expand the definition of iatrogenic to go beyond the medical and include anything in our normal environment that is destructive to the individual. Looked at in this way, we can see that humans are well on the way to making the earth an iatrogenic planet, a planet of death.

Human survival is much retarded and aging is accelerated by the accumulated consequences of human evolution. To illustrate my point, let me tell you a little story:

~

It was hard to accept the reality of the man who sat before them. Strapped to a chair, electrodes and electronic probes covering his green body, this was the most important and most secret grilling a captive had ever received. The President spoke: "Mr. Clover, you are the first flying saucer captain we have ever secured. But we are prepared to treat you in a completely humane and dignified manner, befitting your extraordinary diplomatic status. The probes confirm that you are telling us the truth about your age. You are 120 of our earth-solar years, yet you have been body-age tested at 20. The doctors and scientists confirm that. Aside from your unusual skin pigment, you are totally human in all respects. It is clear therefore that you have the secret to lasting life: a pill, an elixir, an operation? ... You have responded to our requests for the secret of your longevity by truthfully discussing Positive attitudes, special diets and meaningful work. Yet the computers say that none of these are enough to account for the amazing degree of youthfulness apparent in a man of your age. They suggest that you are withholding something. Until you disclose that secret, we must keep you incarcerated here on earth. The choice is yours. Please, sir, excuse my bluntness but we insist on candor."

The green man frowned and looked thoughtfully for a moment. Suddenly he burst out laughing. His laugh was infectious and against their will, the military brass, the politicians and the technicians who stood around him began to smile. The green man's booming voice then rang out:

"The question is not why I stay young but rather why you do not. My body age and health are normal for my home planet. Realize that we refer to 'earth' as the death planet. The human contributions to the poisons of your planet have surpassed those of the harsh elements and predatory animals. You continue to increase the background radiation of the atmosphere: a natural age accelerator. You pollute the waters and the air. You attack each other with direct weapons of death: guns, bombs, noise, cars, boredom. You take poisons internally: caffeine, tobacco/nicotine, alcohol, overdoses of salt, refined sugar and cola. You create a psychologically poisonous atmosphere of social stress and competition. You create powerful self-fulfilling social prophecies of premature aging and early death. Your children are raised to value the things most likely to terminate their existence prematurely. We look upon your ice cream parlors, night club bars, candy machines, coke and coffee rituals as the means of slow suicide. What the poisons in the atmosphere do not accomplish quickly enough, you accomplish for yourselves and for your children with Easter baskets, Halloween treats and numerous coffee breaks. You are like lemmings. Some of our philosophers say this is a built-in correction to overpopulation. Some of our historians say this is a consequence of us having used this globe as a prison planet 8,000 years ago: we see here self-flagellation in the hope of regaining access to the beautiful gardens of our home planet: Eden. Whatever the underlying reasons, you are your own victims. Here then is my last secret for youth and longevity: compared to you ... I don't *live* here!"

The probes reflected that all that had been said was honest. The President nodded somberly. He signaled the technicians to release their captive. Lost in thought, he popped a handful of jelly beans into his mouth and then lit up a kingsize filter tip...

~

Growing Younger

The conflict between the pro-longevity people (who believe in a long, youthful life) and the apologists (who accept the status quo and resist attempts at great longevity) is centuries old. The apologists, dominant in most societies, provide a philosophical rationale for maintaining our dubious status as an increasingly suicidal species. Gerontologists, and other scientific visionaries committed to changing human existence for the better, must deal with this mentality head on. My own bias, as you may know by now, is against postnatal abortion ... even if it is "normal" or post-retirement.

Let's look at a few examples of iatrogenic processes active in today's environment as they might affect aging.

The Institutionalization Factor

The practice of medicine, without psychological services, is costly in money, years and effectiveness. If we add clinical psychology (assuming mind and body are unified) to the normal practice of treating physical disorders, we might go a long way toward better health and longevity for all.

Certain drastic medical procedures such as. lobotomy and shock treatment may create their own iatrogenic syndrome, which could accelerate aging and do accelerate illness. Definitive work on the long-term neurological effects of such procedures remains to be done although the procedures have been used for decades. Body age should be tested at the same time.

Mental institutions generate their own expectations of pathological behavior, which make their residents terrified of leaving them. Old folks' homes also engender iatrogenic expectations; mortality on entering such places is extremely high in the first year, particularly during the first three months. Body-age acceleration measurement might highlight this fact more precisely and, we hope, lead to some change.

Other iatrogenic examples are the defeatism and resistance to cure inherent in the apologist philosophies of bureaucrats. San Francisco's Department of Public Health distributed a weekly bulletin on mental retardation to the public which asserted that "unlike mental disorders, mental retardation is an inevitable, lifelong condition. Therefore, adjustment and acceptance rather than a return to normal functioning is the goal.... A rehabilitation group teaches social graces.... The program reaches about 700 mentally retarded each year." (I should add that the bulletin stating these destructive absurdities was later repudiated by county officials.) The very next county, recognizing that about four of every five retardates are environmentally retarded and can readily be treated, had a thriving program whose goal was the return of the mentally retarded to normal functioning. Such goals usually can be reached. The children in one county were taught improved thinking while in the other, they were being offered ways to accept stupidity with style. Retardates who had been taught to accept their disability as immutable were given therapy to learn to live with it. Was taxpayers' money being paid only to have people adjust to their disorders rather than cure them?

It is regrettable that many, if not most, structured public programs for mental retardation still set as goals only the tranquility and behavioral adjustment of their clients. I believe that only when government officials recognize the importance of attempting to *cure* retardates will the mentally retarded really get a fair shake. Meanwhile, we should stop electing the uncured ones.

Families and Schools

The family and the school are the primary cultural transmission lines for all that is negative as well as positive in our society.

We know that a warm, loving family can be a boon to longevity. Yet, conditions in many families are centered on the death wish. The noted comparative psychologist and animal behaviorist J.P. Scott found that when mice fight, their body temperature is elevated significantly. This, in itself, is an aging accelerator. It is the family that can pass on destructive stereotypes of passivity, internalized aggression and the self hate engendered by racism.

Much of what we now consider to be aging may be a consequence of sedentary inactivity—shunning exercise, the outdoors, and any physical activity. What effect does all this have on aging and the quality of life?

We see children medicated to better fit into school patterns, possibly creating dangerous life-shortening addictions. Schools are necessary for proper development of intelligence, cognitive skills and self-concept. We learned, through a careful field assessment of

Growing Younger

3,000 children shut out of public schools in Prince Edward County, Virginia for four years, that the average intelligence of these children fell into the retarded range, by as much as 30 IQ points compared to the pre-closing levels. Only the very brightest did not need the schools; education is rarely geared to the children who need it most.

We know that the teacher learns more readily than the pupil and that teaching is a superior way to learn. But teachers also pass on to children an expected pattern of aging. More than anything else learned in school, particularly during the first few years, your child will learn to be like the teacher. Remember the teachers' smoking room? Not only were no students allowed in there but any student caught smoking on school grounds was in immediate trouble. What better way to sell cigarettes than to make smoking a desired rite of passage to maturity!

Birth

The Freudian psychoanalyst Otto Rank is credited with expounding the controversial theory that birth is a traumatic process with psychological consequences for the adult personality. Freud and most theorists of the analytical movement thought that Rank had gone too far, but today we are taking a second look at his theory. If babies are delivered in an iatrogenic (destructive) way, then he may well have been correct.

What is destructive about childbirth? Some of the medications used, for one thing. Fetus and infant are very vulnerable.

Particularly in the first months following conception, the baby's neurological system is susceptible to iatrogenic substances such as alcohol, hard drugs, caffeine, tranquilizers and LSD. Clearly, prenatal care of mother and child has much to do with subsequent life and ultimate longevity. Of course, birth itself, as David Cheek has demonstrated, becomes a lifelong memory. To keep this memory from being traumatic we now have birth without violence, the LeBoyer method. This gentle transition may well be the normal one, whereas the warped official variation could prove to be highly iatrogenic.

Since LeBoyer began his work too late to affect many of us, is there anything we can do for ourselves as adults? As ever, the im-

Looking at Mistakes

pact of any new idea is greatest when applied to children, but no adult is beyond help or hope. You can be born again. A religious commercial? Yes and no. Inherent in many religious rituals, baptisms and the like, is the concept of going through birth again, this time in the right way. Primal therapy recreated those early movements and allows people to vent the trauma of birth. Another approach is the "Theta Seminars" movement, originated by Leonard Orr in San Francisco. In these seminars, people are immersed in a tub of hot water, supported by two other "rebirthers." Many experience a pulsing energy; the associations are clearly with the original birth process, this time done properly. Then again, hot baths with the right friends also might help.

How would this approach affect longevity? Orr uses the Theta Seminars specifically to undo birth trauma and conditioned death expectations. He believes that people sleep more than they need to as a consequence of both. His seminars therefore promise that less time will be needed for sleeping and that more time will be available for living. Is it effective or just another con? We don't know yet.

Radiation

Background and man-made radiation (X-rays, fallout, improperly shielded appliances and paints) accelerate the aging process. High-energy radiation is the most potent of all pollutants man has unleashed in the environment; even the modest discontinuance of routine chest X-rays and examination under fluoroscopes has reduced the leukemia rate. The radiochemist at the National Center for Atmospheric Research in Boulder, Colorado, who headed an Air Force research group to investigate atmospheric radioactive fallout, linked cancer and arteriosclerosis to tobacco leaves, coke- and coal-burning ovens, and uranium production plants. Mice exposed to X-ray radiation generally die of cancer tumors. A classic example of radiation producing malignant tumors occurred in a factory in which radioactive materials were used to paint luminous figures on watch dials. The women doing the work moistened the brushes with their lips, and by doing so took in an amount of radioactive material sufficient to produce malignancy in their bones.

Science reporter Linda Clark pinpoints nuclear power, color television, microwave towers, high voltage power lines, medical X-rays and fluorescent lights as radiation hazards. More optimistically, she has reviewed some preventive research and suggests specific intakes to counter the iatrogenic effects of these exposures: extra portions of leafy green vegetables, smooth-skinned fruits, protein, sunflower seeds, dessicated liver, vegetable oils, brewer's yeast, vitamin C, vitamin B complex (especially B6), bone marrow, calcium, magnesium, natural iodine, kelp, lecithin and pectin. She also has developed remedy recipes for accumulated exposure to varied radiations, such as vitamin A for fluorescent light defects. How her proposed treatment, let alone the proposed causes, affect the rate of aging awaits body age testing under controlled conditions. Clearly, a technology more oriented to consumer protection might learn to use electric and electronic instruments in such a way that our lives would not be endangered. New shielding and other protective techniques must be developed.

In addition to causing cancer, radiation causes secondary symptoms such as wrinkling, peeling and hardening of the skin, loss of hair and dizziness. Sounds like old age, doesn't it?

A final word about fluorescent lighting. The normal kind is not full spectrum and deprives users of an essential wave band. For children, this can cause vitamin A and D deficiencies (proper synthesis of A and D is dependent on exposure to full-spectrum lighting) and subsequently can affect their bone structure and eyesight. Fluorescent lighting that is full spectrum (such as that manufactured by Duro-Test Electric) and shielded for radiation has been shown to be better for children's activity, behavior, academic performance and bone structure; the standard cool white fluorescent light produces significantly more hyperactivity. This also could relate to the continual flicker of fluorescents at a high frequency, which may block the normal rhythms of neural functioning. Some children even develop convulsions under such lighting, whereas most adults exposed to it for more than an hour just get headaches or find it difficult or impossible to concentrate. It is amazing how many public facilities such as schools, clinics and court rooms use cool-white fluorescent lighting rather than incandescent or the abundant natural light, fortunately still available.

The Iatrogenic Psychology of Defeatism

Clinicians, at times, make mistakes. When these mistakes are repeated systematically they can be categorized and are amenable to prediction. The study of such errors or behavior may be called iatrogenic psychology. Where such intervention has become ritualized or institutionalized, it deserves credit as a pathological entity in its own right.

~

Dr. *A* is a medical specialist (proctology) with credentials in psychiatry and real estate. He has just completed a thorough examination of Georgia, age 5. Dr. A tells Georgia's parents that their child is suffering from a condition we will call "blight," adding, "I'm sorry to have to tell you this, but blight is an incurable illness with a hopeless prognosis."

Certainly such candor is better than lying or misleading Georgia's parents. Nevertheless, Dr. A has erred on scientific, logical and practical grounds. The very act of making such a pronouncement is a key iatrogenic intervention. Surveys suggest that it is a common one—the labels of "incurable" disorder range from cancer to rabies, from mental retardation to psoriasis, epilepsy, racism, heart disease, schizophrenia, autism and senility.

Dr. A's statement implies that successful treatment is impossible. To imply that success has never occurred *in the past* suggests omnipotent awareness of the technological rise and fall of civilization; to imply that it has not occurred in *the present* suggests omnipotent awareness of ongoing treatment across the globe, and to imply that it will never occur *in the future* suggests a thorough knowledge of an infinity of possibilities. In effect, Dr. A suggests that no success will ever occur in either Boston or Stockholm, nor has it ever occurred in Cambridge or Auckland, or anywhere else for that matter.

It could be that Dr. A only meant to say that his best guess was that Georgia would not survive the blight. If so, he intended to make a prediction but communicated a certainty. Logically, if Georgia's parents accept his word, failure is a sure thing. In our universe, sure things are most elusive.

Dr. A was wise not to downplay his concern about the seriousness of Georgia's condition so as to protect her and her parents. But as is often the case with terminally ill patients, this approach deprives the client of the right to crucial personal information. Dr. A was also correct to make no false guarantees of success. However, to revise his original statement into a more accurate and helpful one, he might have said: "I don't know how to cure Georgia's blight nor do I know of anyone who can. Based on the most recent statistics I can find, of every hundred children who have contracted the blight only two have survived it. That means, without some treatment of which I'm not aware, your daughter's chances of non-survival are at best 50:1."

This would be a less devastating statement than the one made earlier, but clearly it is not head-in-the-clouds optimism either. The new statement also admits professional limitations and lack of information—an important, but rarely exercised, professional responsibility.

To complete his more thoughtful alternate response, Dr. A might add: "I will, however, immediately do some more reading, consult experts in this area, and get back to you as soon as I have anything new to suggest. In the meantime, I very much recommend that you get a second opinion."

Dr. A is now being honest about his limited awareness of current research. He is open to changing his prognosis if new information comes to light. He has shown a willingness to learn more in the interest of his patient by undefensively recommending a second opinion to validate his own. Dr. A now demonstrates both professionalism and realism, not defeatism or pseudo-omnipotence. As a contemporary pragmatist, he is no longer being negative by implying that "If I can't help you, no one can." Is such a practitioner too good to be true?

Disabling human pathology is under assault throughout the modern world. No disorder stands unchallenged and most seem to have yielded ground to a variety of treatments. As ever, there is a tremendous gap between published breakthroughs and their widespread use. Professional and public education can narrow this gap. Yet, it is not unusual for successful treatment to exist in close proximity to practitioners who are vocal on the incurability of the disorder. Bureaucracies often justify a lack of expenditure on costly but effective innovations by maintaining that an illness is incurable. It is much easier to say that something cannot be done than to grapple honestly with the politically sensitive question of whether or not the expense is worth it. So goes the socially iatrogenic impact of the defeatist practitioners and researchers; yet, some of the most prestigious gladly accept huge sums of research money to solve problems they have already categorized as hopeless.

The Distinguished Scientist Surveys

To illustrate my own ideas about iatrogenic defeatism, I sent a series of surveys to 370 psychologists, psychiatrists and physicians, randomly selected from their national association directories. I gave them the opportunity to submit examples of "incurable" disorders. Despite the practical absurdity of identifying anything as "incurable," the majority of the 139 who replied did exactly that, often listing disorders relevant to their own specialty as hopeless. To the extent that the respondents were representative of clinical practice, my guess is that scientifically grounded non-defeatist practitioners include one of every two psychologists, one of every four psychiatrists and one of every ten non-psychiatric physicians.

Fifty-one percent of the psychologists wrote back naming incurables. Of the 79 disorders listed, many were commonly-diagnosed mental disorders including "schizophrenia," "mental retardation," "autism," "senile psychoses," "trauma-induced mental aberration" and "mental illness." Other, presumably nonorganic, incurables were "stupidity" and "white racism." Of the 64 predominantly organic diagnoses, most of the "incurable" labels were pinned on "cancer" and "heart disease," as might have been expected. Others named "neurological diseases," "arthritis," "muscular dystrophy" and "physical disorders of aging." "Epilepsy," "crib deaths," "rabies," "diabetes" and "psoriasis" received one vote each.

From the nearly half who did not choose to suggest any incurable disorders, I received many calm but forceful lectures on the philosophy and logic of science: "You cannot demonstrate that a disease is incurable: only that it is curable," and "I don't like the term 'incurable': it implies an absolute." Some expressed sentiment: "I feel no human illness is potentially incurable" (leaving nonhumans in limbo). Others modestly stressed their limits: "To my knowledge no human illness is incurable." Many requested a definition of terms: "Without a definition of incurable, I cannot judge any human illness as such." There were those who relied on faith: "I am unwilling to believe that any illness is incurable." Then there was the inspirational reply: "Were we, as a nation, to dedicate ourselves to commitment to medical research we should ultimately find cures, I believe, for all that plagues mankind... .

In contrast, one of the most pessimistic contributors to my list of incurable disorders asserted that "every disease is incurable to at least a certain unlucky few, "a sentiment similar in effect to the Buffalonian's saying: "No good deed goes unpunished."

I immediately launched a second survey to poll physicians in every major specialty including psychiatry. Seventy-five percent of the psychiatrists chose to assert the existence of incurable disorders; so did 91% of other specialists.

About one-fifth of the supposedly incurables were mental disorders. When it came to listing the incurables, the psychiatrists were not much different from the psychologists. The other physicians listed significantly more organic incurabies than the psychiatrists or the psychologists, usually in their own area of specialization.

The physicians' responses generally followed those of the psychologists in content, although they plugged more of their self-authored books. Some began positively but shifted gears midway: "I know of no illness that is 100% incurable—by the above I mean that is always incurable—I am excluding the following. .. ." Another could not restrict himself to only three incurables, adding "and many, many others—particularly.. .

Some responses sparkled with wisdom: "No disease is incurable for, given the time, the potential for cure is there, be it physical, emotional or philosophical illness. Anyway, the word cure stems from 'to take care of,' Latin *curare,* and so amelioration is as good as cure any day." One respondent took two full handwritten pages to tell me that I was wasting his time.

My second survey also suggested that, compared to the psychologists, an even larger number of psychiatrists and other medical specialists are willing to say that incurable disorders exist, often in their own area of expertise. Yet every disorder named as incurable

Looking at Mistakes

by any respondent has had successful treatments that have been promoted in contemporary publications. We are surrounded by iatrogenic pessimism, even among those who are most knowledgeable or interested in medical and emotional problems.

Abraham B. Bergman, then president of the National Foundation for Sudden Infant Death in New York, was quoted in *Newsweek* magazine as saying that crib death is "neither predictable nor preventable."

Dr. Lauretta Bender, author of the Bender Motor-Gestalt Test and for many years Chief Psychiatrist at New York's Bellevue Hospital, was an outspoken advocate of shock treatment for children. She asserted that "schizophrenia may be treated but not cured," reporting that a study of her own patients over the years had found none of them to have been helped in a lasting way. Such overgeneralization matches that of the biostatistician who, after a summer night in a cabin filled with "No Pest" strips, decided to declare the mosquito an endangered species.

Mortality and Aging

Doubling your life span is not impossible, but without basic changes in the lifestyle of most of us it is highly improbable.

However, death probabilities have too often been taken as fixed. Leonard Hayflick, a distinguished Stanford microbiologist, discovered that human embryo cells in a test tube subdivide 50 times and no more. Older tissues have fewer divisions. In his much-publicized work over the last decade he has concluded that a biological "clock" determines the speed of cell division and aging. Professional defeatists seized upon Hayflick's research as clear evidence that the maximum human life span, reflected in the limit of 50 cell divisions, was immutable, indicative of built-in limits, perhaps God-given and never to be transcended. Those arguing this way were to some extent successful in arranging funding priorities in age research in such a way that the extension of longevity was unlikely to be financed. Then, as is typical of the history of science, the clear limit we supposedly cannot exceed was exceeded. First, hydrocortisone was used to extend the number of cell doublings by 30 to 50%. Next, a team of Berkeley scientists more than doubled the number of cell divisions by adding an antioxidant, vitamin E, to the culture.

Even at the 97th doubling, 95% of the cells were still viable (able to synthesize DNA); vitamin E had also protected these cells against stress induced by visible light or high-oxygen tension. If the analogy holds, longevity can be doubled by proper dosage of hydrocortisone or vitamin E. (Obviously, this would have to be very carefully tested on humans as well as tissue in test tubes.) To declare a limit to progress is perhaps a catalyst for exceeding that limit.

For decades now, we have had a practical method for testing the individual rate of human aging. With this and related procedures, the specific impact of various stresses, nutrients, therapies and other interventions on human individuals can be evaluated.

Child Development Norms

Until recently, the assertion of the status quo had its place in American psychology. Unfortunately, this assertion, though no longer dominant, still retards our understanding of behavior. Often, those psychologists trained in child development prior to 1950 were taught that the infant's cortex was "nonfunctional" and would remain that way for two years, independent of the environment. Much environmental retardation was supported by this, a self-fulfilling prophecy of sorts. (I once had the delightful experience of bringing my one-year-old to class to argue the point with such a "nonfunctional" psychologist.) How did this destructive interpretation evolve? Decades ago, careful behavioral studies were made of small groups of American children. The observed behavior of each age group was assumed to be normal behavior (or "norms") for American children. Not much attention was paid to how representative these children were of all American children, since it was assumed that every member of a species was much like the others. The norms were seen as biological guidelines describing what a child can do at a given age. Cultural and home environment influences were considered ineffective in changing these biologically-based abilities of infants.

Today, of course, we realize that these norms are primarily a reflection of culture and environment,, genetic and other individual differences being much broader than originally anticipated. Let us briefly examine a few valuable child-based tests in current use: the Bayley Scales of Infant Development, the Vineland Social Maturity Scale, and the Pre-School Attainment Record. Some uninformed

Looking at Mistakes

testers still interpret these norms as biologically based behavioral limits rather than ability samples of fairly small groups of children. Nancy Bayley evaluated 1,262 children in her test; Edgar Doll based his Vineland Scale on 62C children. Since both tests were carefully done, they may be useful in estimating what is normal for many children in our culture, but not what is normal for children of every culture, nor what is possible for children of any culture. By using their combined data. expectations in our culture are that a typical child must be:

- 2 years old to hop on one foot and dry own hands.
- 3 years old to wash own hands unaided, throw objects, know own sex, tell own name.
- 4 years old to wash face unassisted, dress self (except tying), count to 4 and catch.
- 5 years old to blow nose, copy triangle, know own age, name colors.
- 6 years old to use table knife for spreading, bathe self assisted, color drawings, go to bed unassisted.
- 7 years old to ride play vehicles.
- 8 years old to bathe self unaided, use table knife to cut.
- 14.95 years old to communicate by letter.

Those of you who have traveled to places such as Mexico or Hong Kong and have been beguiled by 3-year-old flower sales-girls know that human children can learn to blow their own noses before they are 5, catch a ball before they are 4, know their own sex and name and throw things before they are 3! In Bali, children of 3 may be accomplished musicians of a year or two's experience. What we have here are the norms of children whose development is, on the average, far less than what it could be. Perhaps our self-fulfilling fantasies of helpless infancy have held back our children. But the relative cultural disadvantage illustrated above is not the issue here. The issue is that the role of assessment is to chart progress, not limit it according to preconceived "reality." High school students have been known to be volleyed like ping pong balls between psychologists who push them to fantasize about their careers and guidance counselors who push them to control their fantasies and choose careers that suit their limitations. One can now earn a living either by helping people transcend their limits or by having them accept their limitations.

Cortical Decay

Another example of the frustration of the search for immutable realities can be found in research on the aging of the brain. A basic limitation to the credibility of the cell division studies as an analog of aging is the fact that some cells do not reproduce even once in our life span. Among the most crucial of these are the neurons, building blocks of our brain and the entire nervous system. Most introductory physiology and psychology texts report that once past middle age, one's brain weight decreases with age; and that this reflects progressive loss of nerve cells. The nerve cells, not being able to reproduce, are not replaced. Biostatisticians calculate weight-loss curves and then conclude that, if the rate of loss remained constant, there would be little brain left to see long-lived adults through a second century (although cell loss would not be enough to create serious damage in our present life-span This, then, again seems to put a limit on how long we can expect to extend life.

Assuming this were so, we would still have the potential t develop ways for neurons to reproduce. Another approach would be to find methods to diminish the rate of decay, constancy being the substance of the dismal predictions for great longevity. We're already aware of ways to speed up this decay through drugs alcohol, radiation, stress, etc. If these negative factors, so common in our culture, can promote the decay of neurons perhaps we should blame them on our noxious environment and not consider decay a biological necessity.

Let us look at the basis of the claim that brain weigh decreases with age. While autopsies on humans demonstrate that brain weight has decreased, they cannot indicate the rate of decay when it occurred or even why. Only through careful studies o animals and humans in the last few years have we learned that, in fact, the greatest amount of brain cell death occurs from birth t maturity and not during adult life! This might be due to the greater vulnerability of youth to the accelerators of cortical decay, which may be masked by the ongoing growth processes of childhood. What of the lesser decay that takes place in adult life? Animals in properly protected environments show very little of it as adults. We can now conclude that the decay rate can be slowed by changes in the environment, that children are the most vulnerable to neuron deaths, and that any serious longevity program must recognize that a fully functional brain needs special interventions from infancy on.

Research and Practice in Human Genetics

Nathan Shock, a famous cataloguer of aging research, was once quoted as saying that he could guarantee that our present maximum life span will not be doubled or tripled by any scientific breakthrough because such an increase would violate the genetic code that determines our life span. This rationale was a very common way of looking at aging. Philosophically, it reflects an oft-stated view: "We will die when our number is up and there is little we can do about it except leave the scene with dignity." Not only is this a defeatist philosophy; it is poor genetics, as well. In contrast, Dr. Lissy Jarvik, one of the most important living pioneers of the study of genetics and aging, has this to say:

> It is a common fallacy to assume that because a condition is genetically determined, it is unalterable and incurable. Nothing could be farther from the truth. Actually, if we can demonstrate the hereditary transmission of a condition, a search for its biological correlates is bound to be eventually successful. Once a cause has been determined it can be altered. Indeed the area of mental deficiency provides the example par excellence of how knowledge of genetic factors has enabled us to interfere and to prevent intellectual deficits in individuals genetically predisposed toward them. ... Phenylketonuria, a form of mental deficiency based on the inherited inability to metabolize the amino acid phenylalanine, can now be prevented in most cases by judicious dietary management from earliest infancy.... The attitude of hopelessness, when it comes to aging, is not only unwarranted but has probably been the greatest impediment to progress in the field. It has resulted in restricted financing of research, in a lack of interest on the

part of the young—except for those in our few gerontology centers—and in an attitude of self-deprecation on the part of the aged themselves.

New Directions

Because many new and important approaches can be taken, we must attempt to do what surveys and distinguished scientists have told us was impossible to do.

Guided imagery, which is psychological in nature and can be used to combat cancer, is an example of a promising assault on what is commonly thought to be an "incurable" human ailment. By the same token, hypnosis techniques as developed by such leaders as David Cheek and Leonard Elkind must be applied to attack the problems of aging, birthing, bleeding and, more positively, to enhance the mental abilities of all of us.

Those who hold the purse strings for research and treat.ment, as well as those who contribute to them, must not continue to be overwhelmed by the iatrogenic impact of defeatism. Equally important, the training of future scientists or clinicians should not be led by those whose professional reputations rest on emphatic assertions of limits.

A classic early study most relevant to the iatrogenic psychology of practitioners' defeatism concerned fighting mice who suffered rigged defeats in early adulthood. The study demonstrated that these mice no longer responded to fight training and persisted in their retreat from other mice even after a two-month rest. Subsequently, researchers who have studied a wide variety of species (including ours) have demonstrated that success is less likely after defeats have occurred in early childhood or even adulthood. Speech enables our own species to suffer defeat experienced, or even anticipated, by others.

Aging and its assessment continue to employ both people who spend their professional lives setting limits to progress and those who exceed these limits. Perhaps negative thinking is useful at times, but is it not more difficult to row the boat when someone has dropped anchor?

~12~
Looking at
THE FUTURE
The Phoenix Lodge

THOSE OF US who are convinced that we have only one life to live usually are interested in living it fully. We prefer not to shorten it prematurely, and would like to remain youthful and effective throughout.

Gerontology accumulates new knowledge about life all the time. The information derived from the study of aging has been applied in a piecemeal fashion in various programs across the globe. Insights have been absorbed by many institutions, often without giving credit to gerontology. An example would be the increased popularity of physical fitness testing and training for workers in sedentary jobs. The University of Colorado's physical education department recently set up such a program for its 5,000 faculty and staff members on campus. After using treadmills, health exams and training techniques, workers were found to be more effective at their jobs and to have more positive attitudes. When they are properly tested, we may find that their aging has diminished.

The next step will be to develop therapeutic programs for individuals who want to monitor and change their rate of aging. We may then begin to see the formation of new living patterns based on an anti-aging philosophy.

Legislators now are beginning to respond to the retired voters who, as a result of their increasing numbers and power, are now lobbying against forced retirement.

Deprogramming self-defeating stress and emotional conflict, defusing destructive self-fulfilling prophesies, enhancing personal energy and even lowering body temperatures could all work against premature aging and early death. We can expect to see these and other, perhaps less dramatic, techniques employed by physicians, psychologists, nutritionists and other professionals More and more, people will have the opportunity to choose whether or not to live a full 140 years instead of the average ~0, or to die very prematurely at 35.

If I were developing a program for adults who wished to slow-down or reverse their aging process I would follow these steps:
1. A complete health exam, medical and dental evaluation.
2. A complete psychological exam focused on life and job satisfaction, and career opportunities.
3. A body age test with the Adult Growth Examination.
4. Clients collecting data for a week, writing down everything they eat and drink (including gum and pop, as well as cigarettes smoked) and describing stresses and successes.
5. At the next meeting the test results and the clients' collected data would be examined. An anti-aging program would be devised in which clients would set their own goals for body age and desired length of life.
6. From here on, treatment would include hypnosis, nutritional and psychological interventions. Clients would return each month for a full year to undergo at least one body age test and a review of the anti-aging program. Core body temperatures would also be recorded. The clients would regularly monitor their own diets and levels of satisfaction.

I envisage most of my clients being pre-retirement adults. While people of any age could potentially benefit from anti-aging intervention, I believe that the younger the client, the more promise exists for change. Even children have critical aging periods. In general, private-practice gerontologists would work with adults aged 35 and over. Personally, I would like to concentrate on women moving into their 40s and men into their 50s, since it appears that these are the decades of greatest potential aging, in the absence of treatment.

Good private practice will eventually get around to prevention. This means communicating basic anti-aging principles to all people, whether or not they are paying clients. It also means integrating these concepts into the child-rearing and adult-living patterns of a culture.

Looking at the Future

Newly-emerging lifestyles are rarely absorbed instantly or en masse by a culture. Rather, we may see small groups of initiators living in experimental ways which may or may not prove to be acceptable or successful for everyone. We might envision a "Phoenix Lodge," a model of utopian speculation that initially would be funded by foundations, individuals or cooperatives. This lodge would be a large home or group of homes built for the maximum psychological and social satisfaction of its residents. It would be located at a reasonably high altitude and be fairly isolated. The air would be fresh and no large manufacturing plant or source of radiation would be nearby. We might imagine an extended family as in Robert Heinlein's *Stranger in a Strange Land,* or a communal effort such as the Skinnerian community of Twin Oaks, Virginia.

The diet at the lodge would be devoid of anti-aging components (no cigarettes, no refined sugar, no alcohol, etc.), similar to the one recommended in Nate Pritikin's program. It would contain all the vitamin/mineral benefits described in Michael Lesser's *Nutrition and Vitamin Therapy.* Breakfast would be the large meal of the day and the only one with any bulk. Lunch and supper would be light; both these meals would include liquids (soups and juices), roughage and fruits. A variety of special liquid ambrosias would be developed for children.

The daily routine would include lessons in auto-hypnosis, the martial arts, meditation and other human potential techniques. The birth of a new member would be a community event, well attended and of great importance to everyone.

The residents of Phoenix Lodge would master time acceleration, biofeedback and other techniques to help them choose their own life expectancy and aging rate. The community would be self-sufficient and dynamic, but not totally isolated from the culture surrounding it. Children, all gifted, would become fully independent members by age 10 and, just as the adults, would spend regular periods of their time (perhaps six months every other year) away from the lodge in the larger culture. Personal and community growth would be the natural focus of daily existence.

What would result? One might expect each resident to become a "Phoenix," each day reborn from the ashes of yesterday, living life more fully and consciously than ever before.

Growing Younger

Two things might happen: either the lodges would not effectively relate to the larger culture, and therefore might be envied or destroyed; or, society might follow their lead. If, however, the larger culture were to deteriorate (through a war, for instance), then there might be a tendency to deify and mystify the lodges as well as the people who inhabit them. (They would obviously be stronger, larger, longer-lived, and possess abilities not enjoyed by others.)

Has this happened before in human history? Mount Olympus was 11,000 feet high...

Right now such utopian speculation is only science fiction. We know neither our distant past nor our immediate future. The concept of the Phoenix Lodge is one way to apply as a lifestyle what we have discovered. Can we do better?

Ask yourself first what you *will* do to change your aging and, second, what you would *like* to do. Let your imagination take you to the most relaxing and satisfying place possible, not just for a vacation, but for life. As you continue to make choices about how you live, I hope this book will help you recognize the many that you already have made, as well as some you still wish for.

BIBLIOGRAPHY

Suggested additional readings and complete citations for works referred to in this book.

Aaronson, B.S. Behavior and the place names of time. *American Journal of Hypnosis: Clinical, Experimental, and Theoretical,* 1966, 9, 1—17.

Aaronson, B.S. Hypnotic alterations of space and time. *International Journal of Parapsychology,* 1968a, *10,* 5—36.

Aaronson, B.S. Hypnosis, time rate perception, and personality. *Journal of Schizophrenia,* 1968b, *2,* 11—41.

Abrahamson, E.M. and Pezet, A.W. *Body, mind, and sugar.* New York: Pyramid, 1971.

Abrams, A., Tobin, S.S., Gordon, P., Pechtel, C., and Hilkevitch, A. The effects of a European procaine preparation in an aged population. I. Psychological effects. *Journal of Gerontology,* 1965, *20,* 139—143.

Adams, R. and Murray, F. *Megavitamin therapy.* New York: Pinnacle, 1975.

Adaptation of the Denver Development Screening Test. *Today's Health,* September, 1972, *50,* 35.

Alexander, F. *Psychosomatic medicine.* New York: Norton, 1950.

American Heart Association. Major rise factors in heart disease. *World Almanac and Book of Facts 1976.* New York: Newspaper Enterprise Association, 1975.

Aslan, A. Theoretical and practical aspects of chemotherapeutic techniques in the retardation of the aging process. In M. Rockstein, M. Sussman, and J. Chesky (Editors) *Theoretical aspects of aging.* New York: Academic Press, 1974, pp. 145—156.

Baltes, P.B. Longitudinal and cross sectional consequences in the study of age and generation effects. *Human Development,* 1968, *11,* 145—171.

Barber, T.X. *LSD, marijuana, yoga, and hypnosis.* Chicago: Aldine, 1970.
Barber, T.X. *Hypnosis: a scientific approach.* New York: Van Nostrand-Reinhold, 1969.
Barrett, J.H. *Gerontological Psuchology.* Sprir₁gfield, Illinois: Thomas, 1972.
Barrows, C.H. and Beauchene, R.E. Aging and nutrition. In A.A. Albanese (Editor) *Newer methods of nutritional biochemistry,* Volume 4. New York: Academic Press, 1970.
Bayley, N. *Manual for the Bayley Scales of Infant Development.* New York: Psychological Corporation, 1969.
Beard, R.E. Note on some mathematical mortality models. In G.E.W. VVolstenholme and M. O'Connor (Editors) *The lifespan of animals,* Volume 5. Boston: Little, Brown, & Company, 1959, 302-311.
Beech, H.K. Nonspecific forces surrounding disease and the treat ment of disease. *Journal of the American Medical Association,* 1962, *179* 437-440.
Bellamy, D. Long term action of prednisolone phosphate on a strain of short—lived mice. *Experimental Gerontology,* 1968, *3,* 327—333.
Beller, S. and Palmore, E. Longevity in Turkey. *The Gerontologist,* 1974, *14,* 373—376.
Belsky, J. *The Adult Experience.* San Francisco: West/Wadsworth, 1997.
Bender, A.D., Kormendy, C.G., and Powell, R. Pharmacological control of aging. *Experimental Gerontology,* 1970, *5,* 97—129.
Bender, L. Alpha and omega of childhood schizophrenia. *Journal of Autism and Childhood,* 1971, *1,* 115—118.
Benet. S. *How to live to be 100.* New York: Dial, 1976.
Benet, S. *Abkhasians: the long-living people of the Caucasus (Case studies in cultural anthropology).* New York: Holt, Rinehart, & Winston, 1974.
Benet, S. Why they live to be 100, or even older, in Abkhasia. *The New York Times Magazine,* 1971, December 26.
Benjamin, H. Outline of a method to estimate the biological age with special reference to the role of sexual functions. *International Journal of Sexology,* 1949, *3,* 34—37.

Bentler, P.M. and Hilgard, E.R. A comparison of group and individual induction of hypnosis with self-scoring and observer-scoring. *International Journal of Clinical and Experimental Hypnosis,* 1963, *11,* 49—54.

Berg, B.N. and Simms, H.S. Reduced caloric intake in rats does not need stunting of growth or blocked sexual maturation to be effective. *Journal of Nutrition,* 1960, *71,* 255.

Bergman, A.B. Crib death. *Newsweek,* September 3, 1973, *82,* 12.

Bernstein, F. Law of physiological aging as derived from long range data in refraction of the human eye. *Archives of Ophthalmology,* 1945, *34,* 378-388.

Bindra, J.S. Anti-aging drugs. In R.V. Heinzelman (Editor) *Annual reports in medicinal chemistry,* Volume 9. New York: Academic Press, 1974, 215—221.

Bird, C. LeBayer follow-up, *New Age Journal,* 1975 (November), 14-15. Birren, J.E. (Editor). *Relations of development and aging.* Springfield, Illinois: Thomas, 1965.

Birren, J.E. *The psychology of aging.* Englewood Cliffs, New Jersey: Prentice-Hall, 1964.

Birren, J.E. A brief history of the psychology of aging. I and II. *The Gerontologist,* 1961, *1,* 67—77 and 127—134.

Birren, J.E. Psychological aspects of aging. *Annual Review of Psychology,* 1960, *11,* 161—198.

Birren, J.E. (Editor) *Handbook of aging and the individual: psychological and biological aspects.* Chicago: University of Chicago Press, 1959.

Birren, J.E., Butler, R.N., Greenhouse, S.W., Sokoloff, L., and Yarrow, M.R. Human aging: a biological and behavioral study, U.S. Public Health Service Publication No. 986. Bethesda: National Institute of Mental Health, U.S. Department of Health, Education, and Welfare, 1963.

Birren, J.E. and Fox, C. Accuracy of age statements by the elderly. *Journal of Abnor- mal and Social Psychology,* 1950, *45,* 384—387.

Birren, J.E., Imus, H.A., and Windle, W.F. (Editors). *The process of aging and the nervous system.* Oxford: Blackwell Scientific Publications, 1959.

Birren, J.E.; Kenyon, G.M.; Ruth, J. editors. *Aging & Biography: Explorations in Adult Development.* New York: Springer Pub. Co., 1996.

Birren, J.E., Riegel, K.F., and Morrison, D.F. Age differences in response speed as a function of controlled variations of stimulus conditions: evidence of a general speed factor. *Gerontologia,* 1962, *6,* 1—18.

Birren, J.E. and Schaie, K.W. (Editors). *Handbook of the Psychology of Aging.* New York: Van Nostrand Reinhold, 1977.

Birren, J.E. and Spieth, W. Age, response speed, and cardiovascular functions. *Journal of Gerontology,* 1962, *17,* 390—391.

Birren, J.E. and Wall, P.D. Age changes in conduction velocity, refractory period, number of fibers, connective tissue space and. blood vessels in sciatic nerve of rats. *Journal of Comparative Neurology,* 1956, *104,* 1—16.

Bischof, L.J. *Adult psychology, second edition.* NewYork: Harper & Row, 1976.

Bjorksten, I. The cross-linkage theory of aging. *Journal of the Geriatric Society,* 1968, *16,* 408—427.

Bligh, I. *Temperature regulation in mammals and other vertebrates.* New York: American Elsevier, 1973.

Bockoven, 1.5. Aspects of geriatric care and treatment: moral, amoral, and immoral. In R. Kastenbaum (Editor). *New thoughts on old age.* New York: Springer, 1964, 213-225.

Bolgen, K. No hopeless children. *The Humanist,* 1970 (July/August), 14-22.

Bortz, W.M. and Bortz, E.L. Race and differential aging. *Hawaii Medical Journal,* 1956, *16,* 134—175.

Botwinick, I. *Aging and behavior.* New York: Springer, 1973.

Botwinick, I. Geropsychology. *Annual Review of Psychology,* 1970, *21,* 239-272.

Botwinick, I. A crude test of a hypothesis relating rate of growth to length of life. The Gerontologist, 1968, *8,* 196—197.

Boucher, R.G. and Hilgard, E.R. Volunteer bias in hypnotic experimentation. *American Journal of Clinical Hypnosis,* 1962, *5,* 49—51.

Bourliere, F. Assessing biological age. In P. Williams, C. Tibbitts, and W. Donahue (Editors). *Processes of aging: I.*

New York: Atherton, 1963, 184—197.
Bourliere, F. The comparative biology of aging. *Journal of Gerontology* 1958, Supplement 2, *13*, 16—24.
Bowes, W.A., Brackbill, Y., Conway E., and Steinschneider, A. The effects of obstetrical medication on fetus and infant. *Monographs of the Society for Research in Child Development,* 1970, *35,* 1—55.
Braines, D. Unpublished experiment on canine rejuvenation through reduced metabolic rate during induced sleep. Davidofsky Laboratory, USSR Psychiatry Institute, July, 1957. In DeLaney, R., 1962, Ch. 7.
Brekham, 1.1. *Panax Ginseng—I.* Medical Science and Service. 1967, *4,* 17-26.
Brenman, M. and Gill, M.M. *Hypnotherapy.* New York: International Universities Press, 1947.
Brodie, B.B. and Axelrod, J. The fate of aminopyrene (Pyramidon) in man and methods for the estimation of aminopyrene and its metabolites in biological material. *Journal of Pharmacology and Experimental Therapy,* 1950, 99, 171—184.
Brodine, V. (Editor) *Nuclear information: strontium 90 fallout, baby tooth survey, food fallout, and genetic defects.* St. Louis, Missouri: Greater St. Louis Citizens Committee for Nuclear Information, March 1963.
Brody, H. Structural changes in the aging nervous system. *Interdisciplinary Topics in Gerontology,* 1970, 7, 9—21.
Bromley, D.B. *The psychology of human aging.* Baltimore: Penguin Books, 1966.
Browning, C.W., Quinn, L.H., and Crasilneck, H.B. The use of hypnosis in suppression amblyopia of children. *American Journal of Ophthalmology,* 1958, 46, 53—67.
Bruckner, R. Uber methoden longitudinaler alternforschung am auge. *Ophthalmologica,* 1959, *138,* 59—75.
Buetow, D.E. Cellular content and cellular proliferation changes in the tissues and organs of the aging mammals. In I.L. Cameron and J.D. Thrasher (Editors). *Cellular and molecular renewal in the mammalian body.* New York: Academic Press, 1971, 87—106.
Buhler, C., Keith-Spiegel, P., and Thomas, K. Developmental psychology. In B.B. Wolman (Editor). *Handbook of General Psy-*

chology. Englewood Cliffs, New Jersey: Prentice-Hall, 1973. Chapter 42, 861—917.

Burgess, E.W. A comparison of the interdisciplinary findings of the study of objective criteria of aging. In C. Tibbitts and W. Donahue (Editors). *Social and psychological aspects of aging—aging around the world: Proceedings of the Fifth Congress of the International Association of Gerontology in San Francisco, 1960.* New York: Columbia University Press, 1962.

Burke, D. and Mann, D.F. Influence of several automatic drugs on sodium nitroprusside and oxotremorine-induced hypothermia in immature and mature mice. *Journal of the Pharmaceutical Sciences,* 1970, *59,* 1814—1818.

Burley-Allen, M. Distinguished Scientist Survey III. (Unpublished survey, San Francisco State University, 1974).

Burr, H.S. Blueprint for immortality: the electric patterns of life. London: Neville Spearman, Ltd., 1972.

Butler, R.N. Age: the life review. *Psychology Today,* 1971, *5 (7),* 49.

Cafruny, E.J. Pharmacological intervention of aging process: summary and remarks. *Advanced Experimental Medical Biology,* 1978, 97, 225—230.

Caird, W.K. Memory loss in the senile psychoses: organic or psychogenic? *Psychological Reports,* 1966, *18,* 788—790.

Calder, N. *The mind of man.* New York: Viking Press, 1971.

Cameron, I.L. and Thrasher, J.D. (Editors). *Cellular and molecular renewal in the mammalian body.* New York: Academic Press, 1971.

Campbell, K. Distinguished Scientist Survey II. (Unpublished survey, San Francisco State University, 1973).

Cannon, W.B. Voodoo death. *Psychosomatic medicine,* 1957, *19,* 182—190. Cantor, A.J. *Dr. Cantor's longevity diet.* West Nyack, New York: Parker, 1975.

Carlen, P., Wortzman, G., Holgate, R., Wilkinson, D., and Rankin, J. Reversible cerebral atrophy in recently abstinent chronic alcoholics measured by computed tomography scan. *Science,* 1978, 1076-1078.

Carlson, A.J. and Hoelzel, F. Apparent prolongation of the life span of rats by intermittent fasting. *Journal of Nutrition,* 1946, *31,* 363.

Bibliography

Casey, G.A. Hypnotic time distortion and learning. Unpublished doctoral dissertation, Michigan State University, East Lansing, Michigan, 1966.

Casler, L. Death as a psychosomatic condition: prolegomena to a longitudinal study. *Psychological Reports,* 1970, *27,* 953—954.

Chapanis, A., Garver, W., and Morgan, C.T. *Applied experimental psychology.* New York: Wiley, 1949. (Cf. Chapanis chapter on vision in C.T. Morgan, Editor, *Introduction to psychology,* New York: McGraw-Hill, 1956, 449-479.)

Chebotarev, D.F. and Frolkis, V.V. Research in experimental gerontology in the U.S.S.R. *Journal of Gerontology,* 1975, *30,* 441—447.

Cheek, D.B. Sequential head and shoulder movements appearing with age-regression in hypnosis to birth. *American Journal of Clinical Hypnosis,* 1974, *16,* 261—266.

Cheek, D.B. Communication with the critically ill. *American Journal of Clinical Hypnosis,* 1969, *12,* 75—85.

Cheek, D.B. Further evidence of persistence of hearing under chemoanesthesia: detailed case report. *American Journal of Clinical Hypnosis* 1964, 7, 55—59.

Cheek, D.B. Importance of recognizing that surgical patients behave as though hypnotized. *American Journal of Clinical Hypnosis,* 1962, 227—236.

Cheek, D.B. Unconscious reactions and surgical risk. *Western Journal of Surgery, Obstetrics, and Gynecology,* 1961, 69, 325—328.

Cheek, D.B. Use of pre-operative hypnosis for protection of surgical patients from careless conversation. *American Journal of Clinical Hypnosis,* 1960a, *3,* 101—102.

Cheek, D.B. What does the surgically anesthetized patient hear? *Rocky Mountain Medical Journal,* 1960b, *57,* 49—53.

Cheek, D.B. and LeCron, L.M. *Clinical hypnotherapy.* New York: Grune & Stratton, 1968.

Ciuca, A. and Ghenciu, G. The geography of longevity. *Zeitschrift Alternsforsch,* 1974, *28,* 157—166.

Ciuca, A. and Jucovschi, V. Gerontological research on the organization of services for the elderly. *Gerontologist,* 1973, *13,* 61.

Clark, L. *Are you radioactive?* New York: Pyramid, 1974.

Clark, L. *Stay young longer.* New York: Pyramid, 1961.
Clark, W.G. and Lipton, J.M. Complementary lowering of the behavioural and physiological set-points by tetrodoxin and saxitoxin in the cat. *Journal of Physiology, London,* 1974, *238,* 181—191.
Clarke, J. The aging dimension: a factorial analysis of individual differences with age on psychological and physiological measurements. *Journal of Gerontology,* 1960, *15,* 183—187.
Clemens, J.A. and Fuller, R.W. Chemical manipulation of some aspects of aging. *Advanced Experimental Medical Biology,* 1978, 97, 187—206.
Coburn, A.F., Grey, R.M., and Rivera, S.M. Observations on the relation of heart rate, life span, weight, and mineralization in the digoxin-treated A/J mouse. *Johns Hopkins Medical Journal,* 1971, *128,* 169—193.
Cohen, J. *Psychological time in health and disease.* Springfield, Illinois: Thomas, 1967.
Cohen, Stanley. *Sleep Thieves.* New York: Free Press, 1997.
Comfort, A. Measuring the human aging rate. *Mechanisms of Aging and Development,* 1972, *1,* 101—110.
Comfort, A. *Aging, the biology of senescence.* London: Routledge & Kegan Paul, 1964.
Comfort, A. Test battery to measure aging rate in man. *Lancet,* 1969, *2,* 1411.
Comfort, A. *The process of aging.* London: Weidenfeld & Nicolson, 1965. Cooper, L.F. Time distortion in hypnosis. *Journal of Psychology,* 1952, *34,* 247-284.
Cooper, L.F. Time distortion in hypnosis. *The Bulletin,* Georgetown University Medical Center, 1948, *1* (AprilMay), 214—221.
Cooper, L.F. and Erickson, M.H. *Time distortion in hypnosis.* Baltimore: Williams & Wilkins, 1954.
Cooper. L.F. and Erickson, M.H. Time distortion in hypnosis II. *The Bulletin, Georgetown University Medical Center,* 1950, 4 (Oct/Nov), 50-68.
Cooper, L.F. and Rodgin, D.W. Time distortion in hypnosis and non-motor learning. *Science,* 1952, *115,* 500—502.
Cooper, L.F. and Tuthill, C.E. Time distortion in hypnosis and motor learning. *Journal of Psychology,* 1953, *36,* 67—76.

Corbit,. J.D. Behavioral regulation of body temperature. In J.D. Hardy, A.P. Gagge, and A.J. Stolwijk (Editors). *Physiological and behavioral temperature regulation.* Springfield, Illinois: Thomas, 1970, Ch. *53,* 777-801.

Corday, E. and Vyden, K. Electronic monitors in medicine. *Journal of the American Association of Medical Instrumentation,* 1966, 7.

Corso, J.F. Age and sex differences in pure-tone thresholds. *Journal of the Acoustical Society of America,* 1959, *3 1,* 498-507.

Cosh, J.A. Studies on the nature of the vibrations sense. *Clinical Science,* 1953, *12,* 131—151.

Coué, E. *Self-mastery through conscious autosuggestion (1922).* London: Allen & Unwin, 1951.

Coué, E. *How to practice suggestion and auto-suggestion.* New York: American Library Service. 1923.

Cox, B. (Editor). *The Pyramid Guide: Bi-Monthly International Newsletter.* Lake Elsinore, California: El Cariso Publications, 1972-present.

Coyne, J.M. Hypnotherapeutic conditioning. In B.A. Henker (Editor). *Readings in clinical psychology today.* Del Mar, California: CRM, 1970.

Crasilneck, H.B. and Hall, J.A. Physiological changes associated with hypnosis: a review of the literature since 1948. *International Journal of Clinical Experimental Hypnosis,* 1959, 7, 9—50.

Cristofalo, V. Aging. In J. Lash and J.R. Wittaker (Editors). *Concepts of development.* Stamford, Conn.: Sinauer Association, Inc., 1974, 429—447.

Criswell, J.H. The psychologist as perceiver. In R. Tagiuri and L. Petrullo (Editors). *Person perception and interpersonal behavior.* Stanford: Stanford University Press, 1958.

Crumbaugh, J.C. Aging and adjustment: the applicability of logo therapy and the purpose in life test. *The Gerontologist,* 1972, *12,* 418—420.

Cummings, N.A. The health model as entree to the human services model in psychotherapy. *The Clinical Psychologist, 1975, 29,* Fall, 18—21.

Curry, F.J. Mental retardation program. *Weekly Bulletin, City and County of San Francisco Department of Public Health,* 1971, December 27th, 1.

Curtis, H.J. The nature of the aging process. In E. Bittar and N. Bittar (Editors). *The biological basis of medicine,* Volume 1, New York: Academic, 1968.

Davies, D. A shangri-la in Ecuador. *New Scientist,* 1973, Feb. 1, 236—238.

Davis, A.R. and Rawis, W.C. *Magnetism and its effects on the living system.* Hicksville, New York: Exposition, 1975.

Davison, G.C. and Singleton, L. A preliminary report of improved vision under hypnosis. *International Journal of Clinical and Experimental Hypnosis,* 1967, *15,* 57-62.

Dawson, A.M. and Baller, W.R. Relationship between creative activity and the health of the elderly. *Journal of Psychology,* 1972, *82,* 49—58.

Dean, Ward. *Biological Aging Measurement, 2nd edition.* Los Angeles, CA, Center for Bio Gerontology, 1988.

Deemer, W.L. The power of the t-test and the estimation of required sample size. *Journal of Educational Psychology,* 1947, *38,* 329—342.

DeLaney, R. *Develop knowledge unlimited through transitional sleep.* Lexington, Kentucky: Arts and Science Research Foundation, 1962.

de Sainte Colombe, K. and de Sainte Colombe, P. *Manual of applied graphotherapy (revised edition).* Unpublished manuscript available from the authors, Hollywood, California, 1970.

de Vries, H.A. *Vigor regained.* Englewood Cliffs, New Jersey: Prentice Hall, 1974.

Di Cyan, E. *Vitamin E and aging.* New York: Pyramid, 1972.

Dirken, J.M. The functional age of industrial workers. *Mens en ondernem,* 1968a, *22,* 226—273.

Dirken, J.M. A tentative judgment about the "yardstick" for functional age. *Mens en ondernem,* 1968b, *22,* 342—351.

Dmitriev, A.S. and Kochigina, A. The importance of time as a stimulus of conditioned reflex activity. *Psychological Bulletin,* 1959, *56,* 106—132.

Bibliography

Doll, E. A. *Preschool attainment record.* Circle Pines, Minnesota: American Guidance Service, 1966.

Doll, E.A. *Vineland social maturity scale.* Circle Pines, Minnesota: American Guidance Service, 1965.

Doman, G. *How to teach your baby to read.* New York: Simon & Schuster, 1978.

Doman, G. *Teach your baby math.* New York: Simon & Schuster, 1979. Domey, R., McFarland, R. and Chadwick, E. Threshold and rate of dark adaptation as a function of age and time. *Human factors,* 1960, *2,* 109-119.

Donaldson, T.K. Books: Manual for the Adult Growth Examination. *Long Life,* 1980, 4 (2), #17, 43.

Drori, D. and Folman, Y. The effect of mating on the longevity of male rats. *Experimental Gerontology,* 1971, 14, 363—366.

Duane, A. Accommodation. *Archives of Ophthalmology,* 1931, *5,* 1—14.

Duane, A. Subnormal accommodation. *Archives of Ophthalmology,* 1925, *54, 566—587.*

Dufty, 'Al. *Sugar blues.* New York: Chilton, 1975.

Dunbar, H.F. *Emotions and bodily changes.* New York: Columbia University Press, 1954. Particularly 302—310.

Dunker, T. and Tippit, R. *Live longer through sex.* Hermosa Beach, Cal.: Concord House, 1973.

Dunne, D. *Yoga made easy.* New York: Award Books, 1966.

Duran, Eduardo; Duran, Bonnie. *Native American Postcolonial Psychology.* Albany, New York, State University of New York Press, 1995.

Dworkin, S. and Dworkin, F. *The good goodies: recipes for natural snacks 'n' sweets.* Emmaus, Pennsylvania: Rodal Press, 1974.

Edholm, O.G. and Bacharach, A.L. (Editors). *The physiology of human survival.* New York: Academic Press, 1965

.Edmunston, WE. and Erbeck, J.R. Hypnotic time distortion: a note. *American Journal of Clinical Hypnosis,* 1967, *10,* 79—80.

Eisdorfer, C. and Lawton, M.P. *The psychology of adult development and aging.* Washington, D.C.: American Psychological Association, 1973.

Elkind, L. Effects of hypnosis on the process of aging. Unpublished doctoral dissertation, California School of Professional Psy-

chology, San Francisco, 1972.
Elwin, V. *The Muria and their Ghotul.* London: Oxford University Press, 1947.
Emanuel, N.M. and Obukhova, L.K. Types of experimental delay in aging patterns. *Experimental Gerontology,* 1978, *13,* 25—29.
Epstein, J. and Gerson, D. Studies on aging in nematodes IV. The effect of anti-oxidants on cellular damage and life span. *Mechanisms of Aging and Development,* 1972, *1,* 257—264.
Erickson, M.H. and Erickson, E.M. Further considerations of time distortion: subjective time condensation as distinct from time expansion. *American Journal of Clinical Hypnosis,* 1958, *1,* 83—88.
Erickson, M.H. Hypnotic investigation of psychosomatic phenomena. *Psychosomatic Medicine,* 1943, *5,* 51—58.
Erickson, M.H. Collected writings. In I. Haley (Editor), *Advanced techniques of hypnosis and therapy: the collected writings of Milton H. Erickson.* New York: Grune & Stratton, 1967.
Esdaile, J. *Hypnosis on medicine and surgery.* New York: Julian Press, 1957.
Estabrooks, G.H. *Hypnotism (revised edition).* New York: Dutton, 1957.
Everitt, A.V. and Burgess, I.A. *Hypothalamus, pituitary, and aging.* Springfield, Illinois: Thomas, 1975.
Exner, 0. Statistics of the enthalpy-entropy relationship. 1. The special case. *Collections of Czechoslovakian Chemical Communications,* 1972, *37,* 1425.
Eysenck, H.J. An experimental study of the improvement of mental and physical functions in the hypnotic state. *British Journal of Medical Psychology,* 1941, *18,* 304—316.
Feldberg, W. and Myers, R.D. A new concept of temperature regulation by amines in the hypothalamus. *Nature,* 1963, *200,* 1325.
Ferguson, M. (Editor). *Bra jn/Mind Bulletin: Frontiers of Research, Theory, and Practice.* Los Angeles (P.O. Box 42492, Zip 90042): Interface Press, 1975-present.
Ferguson, M. The brain revolution: frontiers of mind research. N e w York: Taplinger, 1973.
Field, J., Fuhrman, F.A., and Martin, A.W. Effect of temperature on the oxygen consumption of brain tissue. *Journal of Neurophysi-*

ology, 1944, 7, 117.

Fischer, R. Biological time, In J.T. Fraser (Editor). *The voices of time.* New York: Braziller, 1966.

Fisher, R.A. *The design of experiments* (4th ed.). London: Oliver & Boyd 1947.

Fisher, S. An investigation of alleged conditioning phenomena under hypnosis. *Journal of Clinical and Experimental Hypnosis,* 1955, 3, 71-103.

Fisher, S. The role of expectancy in the performance of posthypnotic behavior. *Journal of Abnormal and Social Psychology,* 1954, *49,* 503-507.

Florey, C. and Acheson, R.M. *Blood pressure as it relates to physique, blood glucose, and serum cholesterol.* Washington, D.C.: Public Health Service Pub. 1000, series 11, no. 34, 1969.

Folman, Y. and Drori, D. Effects of social isolation and of female odors on the reproductive system, kidneys, and adrenals of unmated male rats. *Journal of Reproductive Fertility,* 1966, *11,* 43—50.

Fozard, J.L. Predicting age in the adult years from psychological assessments of abilities and personality. *Aging and Human Development,* 1972, *3,* 175—182.

Fraisse, P. *The psychology of time.* New York: Harper & Row, 1963.

Frank, B.S. *Nucleic acid therapy in aging and degenerative disease.* New York; Psychological Library, 1969.

Fraser, J.T., Haber, F.C., and Muller, G.H. *The study of time: proceedings of the first conference of the International Society for the Study of Time in Black Forest, West Germany.* New York: Springer-Verlag, 1972.

Freud, S. *A general introduction to psychoanalysis.* New York: Washington Square Press, 1952.

Freyhan, F.A., Woodford, R.B., and Kety, S.S. Cerebral blood flow and metabolism in psychoses of senility. *Journal of Nervous and Mental Disease,* 1951, *113,* 449—456.

Fried, S.B. & Mehrotra, C.M. *Aging & Diversity.* Washington D.C., Taylor & Francis, 1997, Pb.

Friedenwald, J.S. The eye. In A.I. Lansing (Editor). *Cowdry's problem of aging, 3rd edition.* Baltimore: Williams & Wilkins, 1952.

Furukawa, T., Inoue, M., Kajiya, F., Inada, H., Takasugi, S., Fukui, S., Takeda, H., and Abe, H. Assessment of biological age by multiple regression analysis. *Journal of Gerontology,* 1975, *30,* 422—434.

Galton, F. *Inquiries into human faculty and its development,* 2nd edition. New York: Dutton, 1907.

Garst, C.C. *Blood glucose levels in adults.* Washington, D.C.: Public Health Service publication 1000, series 11, no. 18, 1966.

Gavurin, E.I. and Pockell, N.E. Comparison of bare handed and glove handed finger dexterity. *Perceptual and Motor Skills,* 1963, *16,* 246

Geba, B. *Vitality training for older adults: a positive approach to growing older.* New York: Random House, 1974.

Gienke, E.L. The use of hypnosis in visual correction. *Optometric Weekly,* 1957, *48,* 1797—1800.

Gilbert, J.G. *Understanding old age.* New York: Ronald, 1952.

Glorig, A. and Roberts, J. *Hearing levels of adults by age and sex.* Washington, D.C.: Public Health Service publication 1000, series 11, no. 11, 1965.

Goldberg, E.L., Kliman, G.W., and Reiser, M.F. Improved visual recognition during hypnosis. *Archives of General Psychiatry,* 1966, *14,* 100—107.

Goldfarb, A.I. Predicting mortality in the institutionalized aged, a seven year follow-up. *Archives of General Psychiatry,* 1969, *21,* 172—176.

Gompertz, B. On the nature of the function expressive of the law of human mortality and on a new mode of determining life contingencies. *Philosophical Transactions of the Royal Society (London),* series A. 1825, *115,* 513.

Gordon, H.A., Bruckner-Kardoss, E., and Wostmann, B.S. Aging in germ-free mice: life tables and lesions observed at natural death. *Journal of Gerontology,* 1966, *21,* 380—387.

Gordon, P., Tobin, S.S., Doty, B., and Nash, M. Public Health Service publication 1000, series 11, no. 5, 1964b.

Gordon, T. and Devine, B. *Hypertension and hypertensive heart disease in adults.* Washington, D.C.: Public Health Service publication 1000, series 11, no. 13, 1966.

Gorton, B.E. Current problems of physiologic research in hypnosis. In G.H. Estabrooks (Editor), *Hypnosis: current problems.* New York: Harper & Row, 1962.

Gorton, B.E. The physiology of hypnosis: a review of hypnosis. *Psychiatric Quarterly,* 1949, *23,* 317—343 and 457—485.

Graef, J.R. The influence of cognitive states on time estimation and subjective time rate. Doctoral dissertation, unpublished, at the University of Michigan, Ann Arbor, 1969.

Granick, S. and Patterson, RD. *Human aging II: an eleven year followup biomedical and behavioral study.* Rockville, Maryland: USDHEW National Institute of Mental Health Publication (HSM) 71—9037, 1971.

Green, R.L., Hoffman, L.J., Morse, R., and Morgan, R.F. *The educational status of children during the first school year following four years of little or no schooling.* Washington, D.C.: U.S. Office of Education cooperative research project 2498 report, 1965.

Green, R.L. and Morgan, R.F. The effects of resumed schooling on the measured intelligence of Prince Edward County's black children. In Roger Wilcox (Editor), *The psychological consequences of being a black American: research by black psychologists.* New York: Wiley 1970.

Green, R.L., Morgan, R.F., and Hoffman, L.J. The effects of deprivation on intelligence, achievement, and cognitive growth. In Roger Wilcox (Editor), *The psychological consequences of be ing a black American: research by black psychologists.* New York: Wiley, 1970b. Reprinted from the original 1967 article in the *Journal of Negro Education.*

Greenwood, M. "Laws" or mortality from the biological point of view. *Journal of Hygiene,* 1928, *28,* 267.

Gruman, G.J. *History of Ideas about the Prolongation of Life.* Stamford, N.H., Ayer co. Pub., 1977. (Out of print, but available from instructor.)

Gruman, G. *A history of ideas about the prolongation of life.* (Transactions of the American Philosophical Society, *56,* part 9), New York: Arno, 1977.

Grunbaum, A. The status of temporal becoming. In R. Fisher (Editor) *Interdisciplinary perspectives of time, annals of the*

New York Academy of Sciences. New York: New York Academy of Sciences, 1967, *138,* 374-395.

Gumbel, E.J. *Statistics of extremes.* New York: Columbia University Press, 1958.

Haley, J. (Editor). *Advanced techniques of hypnosis and therapy: the collected writings of Milton H. Erickson.* New York: Grune & Stratton, 1967.

Halsell, G. Mind over cancer. *Prevention,* 1976, *28,* (January), 118—127.

Hamlin, R.M. A utility theory of old age. *The Gerontologist,* 1967, 7, 37-45.

Hamlin, R.M. Utility theory of old age. *Proceedings of the 74th annual convention of the American Psychological Association,* 1966, 213—214.

Hammel, H.T. Regulation of the internal body temperature. *American Review of Physiology,* 1968, *30,* 641—710.

Hardy, J.D. Peripheral inputs to the central regulator for body temperature. In S. Itoh, K. Ogata, and H. Yoshimura (Editors), *Advances in climatic physiology,* Tokyo: Igako Shoin, 1972, 3—21..

Harman, D. Free radical theory of aging: effect of the amount and degree of unsaturation of dietary fat on the mortality rate. *Journal of Gerontology,* 1971, *26,* 451—457.

Harman, D. Free radical theory of aging: relations between antiaging and chronic-radiation protection agents. *Radiation Research,* 1968a, *35,* 547.

Harman, D. Free radical theory of aging: effect of free radical reaction inhibitors on the mortality rate of the male LAFI mice. *Journal of Gerontology,* 1968b, *23,* 476-482.

Harman, D. Prolongation of the normal life span and inhibition of spontaneous cancer by antioxidants. *Journal of Gerontology,* 1961, *16,* 247-254.

Harman, D. Prolongation of the normal lifespan by radiation protection chemicals. *Journal of Gerontology,* 1957, *12,* 257—263.

Harris, M. Temperature, resistant variants in clonal populations of pig kidney cells. *Experimental Cell Research,* 1967, *46,* 301.

Hartland, J. *Medical and dental hypnosis.* London: Bailliere, Tindall, & Cassell, 1966.

Harwood, E. Re-ablement and re-activation for the elderly and dis-

Bibliography

abled. Unpublished paper presented to the South Australian Council on the Aging Geriatric Conference, Adelaide, 1977.
Havighurst, R.J. and Albrecht, R. *Older people.* New York: Longmans, Green, 1953.
Hayflick, L. The longevity of cultured human cells. *Journal of the American Geriatrics Society,* 1974a, *22,* 1—12.
Hayflick, L. The strategy of senescence. *The Gerontologist,* 1974b, *14,* 37—45.
Hayflick, L. Aging under glass. *Experimental Gerontology,* 1970, *5,* 291-303.
Hayflick, L. The limited in vitro lifetime of human diploid cell strains. *Experimental Cell Research,* 1965, *37,* 614—636.
Hebbelinck, M. Kinanthropometry and aging: morphological, structural, body mechanics, and motor fitness aspects of aging. In F. Landry and W.A. Orban (Eds.), *Physical activity and the aging process.* Book 1 of the International Congress on Physical Activity Sciences, Miami: Symposia Specialists, 1978, 95—110.
Heidemann, R. *Presbyopie and Lebensdauer.* Goettinger: Inaugural Dissertation, 1932.
Heinlein, R.A. *Stranger in a strange land.* New York: Avon (Putnams), 1961.
Heldmaier, G. and Hoffmann, K. Melatonin stimulates growth of brown adipose tissue. *Nature,* 1974, *247,* 224—225.
Hemingway, P.D. *The transcendental meditation primer.* New York: Dell, 1976.
Hershey, D. *Lifespan and factors affecting it.* Springfield, Illinois: Thomas, 1974.
Heynen, J. *One Hundren Over 100.* Golden, CO., Fulcrum Pub., 1990.
Hilgard, I. *Personality and hypnosis.* Chicago, Illinois: University of Chicago Press, 1970.
Hilgard, j. *Hypnotic susceptibility.* New York: Harcourt, Brace, & World, 1965.
Hofstetter, H.W. Some interrelationships of age, refraction, and rate of refractive changes. *American Journal of Optometry,* 1954, *31,* 161-169.
Hofstetter, H.W. A comparison of Duane's and Donder's tables of the amplitudes of accommodation. *American Journal of Op-*

tometry, 1944, *21*, 345—363.
Holden, E.M. Primal pain and aging. *Journal of Primal Therapy*, 1974a, *2*, 97-110.
Holden, E.M. The significance of research on vital signs in primal therapy, *Journal of Primal Therapy*. 1974b, *2*, 120—125.
Hollingsworth, D.R., Hollingsworth, J.W., Bogitch, S. Neuromuscular tests of aging in Hiroshima survivors. *Journal of Gerontology*, 1969, *24*, 276—283.
Hollingsworth, J.W., Hashizume, A. and Jablon, S. Correlations between tests of aging in Hiroshima subjects—an attempt to de fine physiologic age. *Yale Journal of Biological Medicine*, 1965, *38*, 11.
Holmes, T. The social readjustment rating scale. *Journal of Psychosomatic Research*, 1967, *2:* in 0. Segerberg, *The immortality factor.* New York; Dutton, 1974, 95.
Holtzman, D., Lovell, R.A., Jaffe, A.H., and Freedman, D.X. 1—Delta—g... Tetrahydrocannabinol: neurochemical and behavioral effects in the mouse. *Science*, 1969, *163*, March: 3874, 1464-1467.
Hrachovec, J.P. *Keeping younger and living longer.* Los Angeles: Sherburne, 1972.
Hutschnecker, A.A. *The will to live.* Englewood Cliffs, New Jersey: Prentice-Hall, 1958.
Inglis, J. Psychological investigations of cognitive deficit in elderly psychiatric patients. *Psychological Bulletin*, 1958, *54*, 197—214.
Jalavisto, E. The role of simple tests measuring speed and performance in the assessment of biological vigour: a factorial study of elderly women. In A. Welford and J. Birren (Editors), *Behavior, aging, and the nervous system.* Springfield, Illinois: Thomas; 1965, 13—25.
Jalavisto, E. and Makkonen, T. On the assessment of biological age: I. Factor analysis of physiological measurements in old and young women. *Annals of the Academy of Fenn. Science*, 1963a, *100*, 1—38.
Jalavisto, E. and Makkonen, T. On the assessment of biological age: II. A factorial study of aging in postmenopausal women. *Annals of the Academy of Fenn. Science*, 1963b, *101*, 1—15.

Bibliography

Jarvik, L. Thoughts on the psychobiology of aging. *American Psychologist,* 1975, *30,* 576-583.

Jeffers, F., Eisdorfer, C., and Busse, E. Measurement of age identification: a methodological note. *Journal of Gerontology,* 1962, *17,* 437-439.

Jewett, S.P. Longevity and the longevity syndrome. *The Gerontologist,* 1973, *13,* 91-99.

Johnson, E.S., Kelly, I.E., and Van Kirk, L.E. *Selected dental findings for adults.* Washington, D.C.: Public Health Service publication 1000, series 11, no. *7, 1965.*

Johnson, H.A. and Pavelec, M. Thermal injury due to normal body temperature. *American Journal of Pathology,* 1972, 66, 557.

Jones, H.B., Gofman, JAN., Lindren, FT., Lyon, T.P., and Strisower, B. Lipoproteins in atherosclerosis. *American Journal of Medicine,* 1951, *11,358—380.*

Jones, H.E. Intelligence and problem-solving. In J.E. Birren (Editor), *Handbook of aging and the individual.* Chicago: University of Chicago Press, 1959, 731—733.

Kahn, S. *Essays on longevity.* New York: Philosophical Library, 1974. Kahn, T.C. Four methods having medical and behavioral diagnostic potential: a proposal. *Perceptual and Motor Skills,* 1964, *18,* 443—444.

Karon, B.P. The resolution of acute schizophrenic reactions: a contribution to the development of non-classical psychotherapeutic techniques. *Psychotherapy: theory, research, and practice,* 1963, *1,* 27—43.

Karon, B.P. and Vandenbos, G.R. Cost/benefit analysis: psychologist versus psychiatrist for schizophrenics. *Professional Psychology,* 1976, 7, 107—111.

Kastenbaum, R. Age: getting there ahead of time. *Psychology Today,* 1971, *5, (7),* 53.

Kastenbaum, R. (Editor). *New thoughts on old age.* New York: Springer, 1964.

Kastenbaum, R., Derbin, V., Sabatini, P., and Artt, S. "The ages of me" toward personal and interpersonal definitions of functional aging. *Aging and Human Development,* 1972, *3,* 197—212.

Kaufman, M.R. Old age and aging: the psychoanalytic point of view. *American Journal of Orthopsychiatry,* 1940, *19,* 73—79.

Kavaler, L. *Freezing point: cold as a matter of life and death.* New York: John Day, 1970.

Kelley, C.R. Psychological factors in myopia. Paper presented at the annual meeting of the American Psychological Association in New York, August 31, 1961.

Kelley, C.R, Psychological factors in myopia. Unpublished doctoral dissertation at the New School for Social Research, New York, 1958.

Kelly, J.E., Van Kirk, L.E., and Garst, C.C. *Decayed, missing, and filled teeth in adults.* Washington, D.C.: Public Health Service publication 1000, series 11, no. 23, 1967.

Kelly, I.E. and Van Kirk, L.E. *Peridontal disease in adults.* Washington, D.C.: Public Health Service publication 1000, series 11, no. 12, *1965.*

Kemeny, C. and Rosenberg, B. Compensation law in thermodynamics and thermal death. *Nature,* 1973, *243,* 400—401.

Kent, S. *The life extension revolution.* New York: Morrow, 1980.

Klebba, A.J., Maurer, J.D., and Glass, E.J. *Mortality trends for leading causes of death: United States 1950-1969.* Rockville, Maryland: US DHEW, (HRA-74-1853) series 20, no. 16, 1974.

Klopfer, W.G. Psychological stresses of old age. *Geriatrics,* 1958, *13,* 529—531.

Kodman, F., Jr. and Pattie, F.A. Hypnotherapy of psychogenic hearing loss in children. *American Journal of Clinical Hypnosis,* 1958, *1,* 9—13.

Kohn, H.T. and Guttman, P.H. Age at exposure and the late effects of rays: survival and tumor increase in CAF mice irradiated at one to two years of age. *Radiation,* 1963, *18,* 348-373.

Kohn, R.R. *Principles of mammalian aging.* Englewood Cliffs, New Jersey: Prentice-Hall, 1971a.

Kohn, R.R. Effects of anti-oxidants on life span of C57BL mice. *Journal of Gerontology,* 1971b, *26,* 378—380.

Kolb, L.C. *Modern clinical psychiatry* (8th edition). Philadelphia: Saunders, 1973.

Kormendy, C.G. and Bender, A.D. Experimental modifications of the chemistry and biology of the aging process. *Journal of Pharmaceutical Science,* 1971, *60,* 167—180.

Kugler, H.J. *Slowing down the aging process.* New York: Pyramid,

1973.
Kunz, P.R. A time to die? *Newsweek,* 1978, March 6.
Landry, F. and Orban, W.A. (Editors). *Physical activity and the aging process.* Book 1 of the International Congress on Physical Activity Sciences, Miami: Symposia Specialists, 1978.
Lansing, A.I. (Editor). *Cowdry's problems of aging, third edition.* Baltimore: Williams & Wilkins, 1952.
Lapin, I.P. and Samsonova, M.L. Apomorphine hypothermia in mice and the influence on it of adrenergic and serotoninergic agents. *Farmakologiya i Toksikologiya, 1968, 31, 563—567;*
Laughingbird. Thank you, I am free and clear: Leonard Orr and Theta House. *New Age Journal,* 1976, March, 34—39.
Leaf, A. *Youth in old age.* New York: McGraw-Hill, 1975.
Leaf, A. Getting old. *Scientific American,* 1973a, *22 9(3),* September, 44-52.
Leaf, A. Every day is a gift when you are over 100. *National Geographic,* 1973b, *143,* January, 93—118.
Leaf, A. Unusual longevity: the common denominators. *Hospital Practice,* 1973c, *8, 75—86.*
LeBoyer, F. *Birth without violence.* New York: Knopf, 1975.
LeCron, L.M. *Self hypnotism: the technique and its use in daily living.* New York: Signet, 1970.
LeCron, L.M. *Experimental hypnosis.* New York: Citadel Press, 1968.
LeFrancois, Guy. *The Life Span, 6th edition.* San Francisco: Wadsworth, 1999.
Lehmann, H.E. Time and psychopathology. In R. Fischer (Editor) *Interdisciplinary perspectives of time, Annals of the New York Academy of Sciences.* New York: New York Academy of Science, 1967, *138,* 798-821.
Leonard, J.N. and Taylor E.A. *Live Longer Now Cookbook.* New York, Grosset & Dunlop, 1977.
Lesser, G.T., Deutsch, S. and Markovsky, J. Aging in the rat: longitudinal cross-sectional studies of body composition. *American Journal of Physiology,* 1973, *225,* 1472—478
Lessor, M. *Nutrition and Vitamin Therapy.* New York: Grove, 1980; Bantam, 1981.

Levitsky, A. Some additional techniques of hypnosis. *American Journal of Clinical Hypnosis,* 1961, *3,* 231—234.
Lew, E.A. High blood pressure, other risk factors, and longevity: the insurance viewpoint. *American Journal of Medicine,* 1973, *55,* 281-294.
Lifschitz, S. Experimental investigations of suggestibility. *Zhurnal Nevropatologii i Psikhiatrii,* 1927, *20,* 317—324.
Linder, F.E. The health of the American people. *Scientific American,* 1966, 214(6), 21-29.
Linder, F.E. *Cycle I of the health examination survey: sample and response.* Washington, D.C.: Public Health Service publication 1000, series 11, no. 1, 1964.
Lindsley, O.R. Geriatric behavioral prosthetics. In R. Kastenbaum (Editor) *New thoughts on old age.* New York: Springer, 1964, 41—60.
Lints, F.A. and Lints, C.V. Relationship between growth and aging in Drosophila. *Nature New Biology (London),* 1971, *229,* 86—88.
Liu, R.K. and Walford, R.L. The effect of lowered body temperature on lifespan and immune and non-immune processes. *Gerontologia,* 1972, *18,* 363—388.
Loomis, E.A. Space and time perception and distortion in hypnotic states. *Personality,* 1951, *1,* 283.
Lovett Doust, J.W., Huszka, L., and Little, M.H. Metabolic control of body temperature in man. *International Pharmacopsychiatry,* 1973, *8,* 239—244.
Luce, G.G. *Rhythms in psychiatry and medicine.* Washington, D.C.: Public Health Service publication no. 2088, 1970.
Luce, G.G. *Longer Life More Joy: Techniques for Enhancing Health, Happiness and Inner Vision.* North Hollywood, CA, Newcastle Publishing Co., 1992.
Luthe, W. (Editor). *Autogenic therapy, six volumes.* New York: Grune & Stratton, 1970.
Luthe, W. Autogenic training: method, research, and application in medicine. In C.T. Tart (Editor) *Altered states of consciousness.* New York: Wiley, 1969.
Luthe, W. Physiological and psychodynamic effects of autogenic training. In B. Stovkis (Editor) *Topical problems of psychother-*

apy, volume III. Basel, New York: S. Karger, 1960.
Lutwak, L. Symposium on osteoporosis: nutritional aspects of osteoporosis. *Journal of the American Geriatric Society,* 1969, *17,* 116...11g
Maciera-Coelho, A. Action of cortisone on human fibroblasts in vitro *Experientia,* 1966, *22,* 390—393.
MacPherson, K. and Schofield, M. Happiness is a warm bed. Unpub.. lished research at Acadia University, Wolfville, Nova Scotia, 1971.
Maj, J. and Pawlowski, L. The hypothermic effect of L-dopa in the rat. *Life sciences,* 1973, *13,* 141—149.
Makeham, W.M. On the law of mortality. *Journal of the Institute of Actuarians,* 1867, *13,* 325.
Martell, E.A. Inhaled radioactive particles and lethal concentration in body tissues: cancer and atherosclerosis from tobacco leaves, coke ovens, coal-burning, and uranium plants. *Prevention,* 1976, *28,* january, 170-171.
Mathis, E.S. *Socioeconomic characteristics of deceased persons.* Washington, D.C.: Public Health Service publication 1000, series 22. no. 9, 1969.
Mayron, L.W., Ott, J., Nations, R., and Mayron, E.L. Light, radiation, and academic behavior: initial studies on the effects of full spectrum lighting and radiation shielding on behavior and the academic performance of school children. *Academic Therapy,* 1974, *10(1),* 33—47.
McAdams, D.P.; DeSt. Aubin, E. editors. *Generativity & Adult Development.* Washington, D.C., APA, 1998.
McCay, C.M. Chemical aspects of aging and the effect of diet upon aging. In A.L. Lansing (Editor) *Cowdry's problems of aging.* Baltimore: Williams & Wilkins, 1952. Ch. 6, 139—200.
McCay, C.M. *Diet and aging.* Vitamins and Hormones, 1949, *7,* 147.
McCay, C.M. Effect of restricted feeding upon aging and chronic diseases in rats and dogs. *American Journal of Public Health,* 1947,37, 521.
McCay, C.M. and Crowell, M.F. Prolonging the lifespan. *Scientific Monthly,* 1934, *39,* 405—414.

McCay, C.M., Crowell, M.F., and Maynard, L.A. The effect of retarded growth upon the length of the life span and upon the ultimate body size. *Journal of Nutrition,* 1935, *10,* 63—70.
McCay, C.M., Maynard, L.A., Sperling, G., and Barnes, L. Retarded growth, life span, ultimate body size, and age changes in the albino rat after feeding diets restricted in calories. *The Journal of Nutrition,* 1939, *18,* 1—13.
McCay, C.M., Pope, F., and Lunsford, W. Experimental prolongation of life span. *Bulletin of the New York Academy of Medicine,* 1956, *32,* 91-101.
McClure, j.A. *Meat eaters are threatened.* New York: Pyramid, 1973.
McConnachie, B. (Editor). *The job of sex: a workingman 's guide to productive lovemaking.* New York: Warner, 1974.
McFarland, R.A., Tune, G.S., and Welford, A.T. On the driving of automobiles by older people. *Journal of Gerontology,* 1964, *19, 190-197.*
Meares, A. *Hypnotherapy: a study in the therapeutic use of hypnotic painting.* Springfield, Illinois: Thomas, 1957.
Metropolitan Life Insurance Company Socioeconomic Mortality Differentials. *Statistical Bulletin of the Metropolitan Life Insurance Company,* 1975, *56,* January, 2—5.
Milne, L.J. and Milne, M. *The ages of life.* New York: Harcourt, Brace & World, 1968.
Miquel, J. and Robinson, K. A test of physiological age in mice. *Experimental Gerontology,* 1978, *13,* 389—396 (and 1976, *II,* 11).
Mixter, G., Delhery, G.P., Derksen, W.L., and Monahan, T. The influence of time on the death of Hela cells at elevated temperatures. In J.D. Hardy (Editor) *Temperature—its measurement and control in science and industry, volume 3, part 3 (Biology and Medicine).* New York: Reinhold, 1963, 177-182.
Mo, S.S. Temporal reproduction of duration as a function of numerosity. *Bulletin of the Psychonomic Society, 1975, 5,* 165—167.
Moore, F.E. and Gordon, T. *Serum cholesterol levels in adults.* Washington, D.C.: Public Health Service publication 1000, series 11, no. 22, 1967.

Bibliography

Moore, G.E. Lymphoblastoid cell lines from normal persons and those with non-malignant diseases. *Journal of Surgi- cal Research,* 1969, *9,* 139—141.

Moreno, J.L. *The first psychodramatic family.* New York: Beacon, 1967. Morgan, C.T. (Editor). *Introduction to Psychology.* New York: McGraw-Hill, 1956.

Morgan, R.F. *Measurement of Human Aging in Applied Gerontology.* Dubuque, Iowa: Kendall/Hunt Publishing Company, 1981a.

Morgan, R.F. *Interventions in Applied Gerontology.* Dubuque, Iowa: Kendall/Hunt Publishing Company, 1981b.

Morgan, R.F. *The ADULT GROWTH EXAMiNATiON (AGE): Manual for a compact standardized test of individual aging. Third edition (revised).* Waterloo, Ontario: Psychology Department, Wilfrid Laurier University, 1981c.

Morgan, R.F. The definitive method for assessing the genetic basis for behavioral differences between the sexes. In J. Senger (Editor) *Individuals, groups, and the organization.* Cambridge, Mass.: Winthrop, 1980, 15—16. Reprinted from the 1968 publication in *Perceptual and Motor Skills, 27,* 90.

Morgan, R.F. *Conquest of aging: modern measurement and intervention.* Second edition. Pueblo, Colorado: Applied Gerontology Communications, 1977a.

Morgan, R.F. The Adult Growth Examination: follow-up note on comparisons between rapidly aging adults and slowly aging adults as defined by body age. *InterAmerican Journal of Psychology,* 1977b *11,* 10—13.

Morgan, R.F. An introduction to applied gerontology. *Long Term Care and Health Services Administration Quarterly,* 1977c, *1,* 168—178.

Morgan, R.F. *The ADULT GROWTH EXAMINATION (AGE): Manual for a compact standardized test of individual aging. Second edition (revised).* Pueblo, Colorado: Psychology Department, University of Southern Colorado, 1976.

Morgan, R.F. Revision of the Diagnostic and Statistical Manual (DSM.. II) by the addition of iatrogenic disorders and the listing of celibacy as a sexual deviation. *Journal of Irreproducible Results,* 1975,21(2), 21.

Morgan, R.F. The *Adult Growth Examination:* validation, analysis, 11 lasting effects of shock treatment on behavior. *Inter-American Journal of Psychology (Revista Interamericana de Psicologia),* 1967b, *1,* no. 4, 251—261.

Morgan, R.F. Temporal conditioning in humans as a function of intertrial interval and stimulus intensity. Dissertation Abstracts, 1966a, *27,* no. 66—6153. From the doctoral dissertation at Michigan State University, East Lansing, 1965.

Morgan, R.F. The *Hawaii Age Test (HAT)* for bodily aging in adults: standardization and reliability of measures. Alias: the effects of rate and duration of consumption of alcoholic beverages on bodily aging. Unpublished research proposal at Hawaii State Hospital, Haneohe, 1966b.

Morgan, R.F. The isolation, description, and treatment of the pathological behavior of ECT-damaged patients. Paper delivered to the Metropolitan Unit In-service Training Conference, Hawaii State Hospital, Kaneohe, January, 1966c.

Morgan, R.F. Note on the psychopathology of senility: senescent defense against the threat of death. *Psychological Reports,* 1965, *16,* 305—306.

Morgan, R.F. A galvanic skin response technique for the sensory evaluation of annelids. *Papers of the Michigan Academy of Science,* 1964a, *50,* 337-342.

Morgan, R.F. The M/I frequencies: a quick and computation free nonparametric method of test item evaluation. *Psychological Reports,*1964b, 14, 723-728.

Morgan, R.F. The adaptational behavior of chicks in a spinning environment. *Psychological Record,* 1964c, *14,* 153—156.

Morgan, R.F. and Bakan, P. Sensory deprivation hallucinations and other sleep behavior as a function of position, method of report, and anxiety. *Perceptual and Motor Skills,* 1965a, *20,* 19—25.

Morgan, R.F. and Bakan, P. Do-it-yourself hallucinations. *Science Digest,* 1965b, *57,* May, 41-43.

Morgan, R.F. and Fevens, S.K. Reliability of the *Adult Growth Examination:* a standardized test of individual aging. *Perceptual and Motor Skills,* 1972, *34,* 415—419.

Bibliography

Morgan, R.F., Ratner, S.C., and Denny, M.R. Response of annelids to light as measured by the galvanic skin response. *Psychonomic Science,* 1965, *3,* 27—28.

Morgan, R.F. and Toy, T. Learning by teaching: a student-to-student compensatory tutoring program and the Educational Cooperative. In J.G. Sherman (Editor) *PSI personalized system of instruction—Forty-one germinal papers: a selection of readings on the Keller Plan.* Menlo Park: Benjamin, 1974, 180-188.

Morgan, R.F. and Toy, T. Learning by teaching: a student-to-student compensatory tutoring program and the educational cooperative; *Psychological Record,* 1970, *20,* 159—169.

Moriyama, I.M. *The change in the mortality trend in the United States.* Washington, D.C.: Public Health Service publication 1000, series 3, no. 1, 1964.

Moulun, R. and Morgan, R.F. Sibling bondage: a clinical report on a parricide and his brother. *Bulletin of the Menninger Clinic,* 1967, *31,* 229—231.

Muhlbock, 0. Factors influencing the life span of inbred mice. *Gerontologia,* 1959, *3,* 177—183.

Muller, C., and Ciompi, L. *Senile dementia.* Berne, Switzerland: Huber, 1968.

Murray, I.M. Assessment of physiological age by combination of several criteria: vision, hearing, blood pressure, and muscle force. *Journal of Gerontology,* 1951, 6, 120—126.

Myers, R.D. Temperature regulation: neurochemical systems in the hypothalamus. In Haymaker, Anderson, and Nanta (Editors) *The hypothalamus.* Springfield, Illinois: Thomas, 1969, Ch. 14.

National Center for Health Statistics, *Volume II—Section 5: Life Tables.* Rockville, Maryland: Public Health Service HRA 75-1104, 1975a.

National Center for Health Statistics, *Vital statistics of the United States 1971, Volume II—Mortality, Part A.* Rockville, Maryland: Public Health Service HRA 75—1114, 1975b.

National Center for Health Statistics, *Vital statistics of the United States 1971, Volume II—Mortality, Part B.* Rockville, Maryland: Public Health Service HRA 75-1102, 1974.

National Center for Health Statistics. *Vital statistics of the United States, 1967, Volume II—Mortality, Part A.* Washington D.C.: US DREW PHS, 1969.

Neill, A.S. *Freedom, not license.* New York: Hart, 1966.

Neill, A.S. *Summerhill: a radical approach to child rearing.* New York: Hart, 1960.

Neugarten, B.L. *Grow old with me! The best is yet to be.* Psychology Today, 1971, *5(7),* 45.

Newman, S.; Ward, C.R.; Smith, T.B.; Wilson, J. *Intergenerational Programs: Past, Present and Future.* Washington, D.C., Taylor & Francis, 1997, Pb.

Nikitin, V.N. Russian studies on age-associated physiology, biochemistry, and morphology: historic description with bibliography. Bethesda, Maryland: Public Health Service publication no. 857, 1961.

Nordus, I.H.; Vandenbos, G.R.; Berg, S.; Fromholt, P. editors. *Clinical Geropsychology.* Washington, D.C., APA, 1998.

Northrop, J.H. Foreword in R.W. Prehoda, *Extended youth.* New York: Putnam, 1968.

Nuttall, R.L. The strategy of functional age research. *Aging and Human Development,* 1972, *3,* 149—152.

Odens, M. Prolongation of the lifespan in rats. *Journal of the American Geriatrics Society,* 1973, *21,* 450—451.

Orme, JE. *Time, experience, and behaviour.* New York: American Elsevier, 1969.

Orme, J.E. Personality, time estimation, and time experience. *Acta Psychologica,* 1964, *22,* 430.

Orme, I.E. Time estimation and personality. *Journal of Mental Science,* 1962, *108,* 213.

Orne, M.T. On the social psychology of the psychological experiment: with particular reference to demand characteristics and their implications. *American Psychologist,* 1962, *1 7,* 776—783.

Orne, MT. The nature of hypnosis: artifact and essence. *Journal of Abnormal and Social Pyschology,* 1959, *58,* 277—299.

Ornstein, RE. *The nature of human consciousness: a book of readings.* San Francisco: Freeman, 1973.

Bibliography

Ornstein, R.E. *The psychology of consciousness.* New York: Viking, 1972. Ostfeld, A.M. and Gibson, D.C. Summary report and selected papers from a research conference on the epidemiology of aging. Bethesda, Maryland: Public Health Service publication *75—711,* 1972.

Ouseley, S.G.J. *Colour meditations.* London: L.N. Fowler & Co., Ltd., 1949.

Packer, L. and Smith, J. Extension of the lifespan of cultured normal human diploid cells by vitamin E. *Proceedings of the National Academy of Sciences,* USA, 1974, *71,* 4763—4767.

Palmore, E. Predicting longevity: a new method. In E. Palmore (Editor) *Normal aging II: reports from the Duke Longitudinal Studies 1970—1973.* Durham, North Carolina: Duke University Press, 1974a.

Palmore, E. (Editor). *Normal aging II: reports from the Duke Longitudinal Studies 1970—1973.* Durham, N. Carolina: Duke University Press, 1974b.

Palmore, E. (Editor). *Normal aging: reports from the Duke Longitudinal Study 1955—1969.* Durham, N. Carolina: Duke University Press, 1970.

Palmore, E. Physical, mental, and social factors in predicting longevity. *The Gerontologist,* 1969a, *9,* 103—108.

Palmore, E. Predicting longevity: a follow-up controlling for age. *The Gerontologist,* 1969b, *9,* 247-250.

Palmore, E. and Jeffers, F. (Editors). *Prediction of life span.* Lexington, Mass.: Heath, 1971.

Parker, P.D. and Barber, T.X. "Hypnosis", task motivating instructions and learning performance. *Journal of Abnormal and Social Psychology,* 1964, *69,* 499—504.

Passwater, R. *Supernutrition: megavitamin revolution.* New York: Dial Press, 1975.

Pauling, L. *Vitamin C and the common cold.* San Francisco: Freeman, 1970.

Pauling, L. Speculations on the future. In V. Cohn (Editor) *1999, our hopeful future.* New York: Bobbs-Merrill, 1956.

Pearl, R. *The biology of death.* Philadelphia: Lippincott, 1922.

Pelton, R.B. and Williams, R.J. The effect of pantothenic acid on longevity of C—57 mice. *Proceedings of the Society of Experimental Biology and Medicine,* 1958, 99, 632.

Peterson, S. *A catalog of the ways people grow.* New York: Balantine, 1971.

Pierce, R.V. *The people's common sense medical advisor, 12th edition.* Buffalo, New York: World's Dispensary Medical Association, 1883.

Pines, M. *Revolution in learning: the years from birth to six.* New York: Harper and Row, 1966.

Polednak, A.P. and Damon, A. College athletics, longevity, and cause of death. *Human Biology,* 1970, 42, 28—46.

Polk, D.L. and Lipton, J.M. Effects of sodium salicylate, aminopyrene, and chlorpromazine on behavioral temperature regulation. *Pharmacology, Biochemistry, and Behavior,* 1975, 3, 167—172.

Pollard, M. and Kajima, M. Lesions in aged germ-free Wistar rats. *American Journal of Pathology,* 1970, 61, 25—36.

Poplin, L. and DeLong, R. Accelerated aging due to enzymatic racemization. *Gerontology, 1978, 24,* 365—368.

Prehoda, R.W. *Suspended animation.* Philadelphia: Chilton, 1969.

Prehoda, R.W. *Extended youth: the promise of gerontology.* New York: Putnam's, 1968.

Prevention. How to live it up and live longer. Emmaus, Pennsylvania: Rodale, 1974.

Pritikin, N. and McGrady, P. *Pritikin Program for Diet and Exercise.* New York: Grosset & Dunlap, 1979; Bantam, 1980.

Pugh, L.G.C.E. High altitudes. In O.G. Edholm and A.L. Bacharach (Editors) *The physiology of human survival.* New York: Academic Press, 1965.

Quint, J. and Cody, B. Pre-eminence and mortality: longevity of prominent men. *Statistical Bulletin of the Metropolitan Life Insurance Company,* 1968, January, 2—5.

Rambo, V.5. and Sangal, S.P. A study of the accommodation of the people of India. *American Journal of Ophthalmology,* 1960, 49, 993—1004.

Rating, A. and Dietz, B. Effect of subchronic treatment with DB—transtetrahydrocannabinol (D8—THC) on food intake, body temperature, hexobarbitol sleeping time, and hexobarbitol

Bibliography

elimination in rats. *Psychopharmacologia,* 1972, *27,* 349—357.
Ratner, S.C. and Denny, M.R. *Comparative psychology.* Homewood, Illinois: Dorsey, 1964.
Reid, A.F. and Curtsinger, G. Physiological changes associated with hypnosis: the effect of hypnosis on temperature. *The International Journal of Clinical and Experimental Hypnosis,* 1968, *16,* 111—119.
Rejuvenation. Published by the International Association on the Artificial Prolongation of the Human Species *Lifespan.* 12 Knokke-Zoute, B—8300, Belgium.
Richardson, M.W. and Stalnaker, J.M. Time estimation in the hypnotic trance. *Journal of General Psychology,* 1930, 4, 362—366.
Richter, C. On the phenomenon of sudden death in animals and men. *Psychosomatic Medicine,* 1957, *19,* 191—198.
Riley, M.L. and Foner, A. *Aging and society: inventory of research findings.* New York: Russell Sage Foundation, 1968.
Riley, M.L., Riley, J.W., and Johnson, M.E. *Aging and society, volume two: aging and the professions.* New York: Russell Sage Foundation, 1969.
Rimmer, R. *The Harrad Experiment.* New York: Bantam, 1967a.
Rimmer, R. *The rebellion of Yale Marratt.* New York: Avon, 1967b.
Robbins, T. *Jitterbug Perfume.* New York: Bantam Books, 1990, Pb.
Roberts, J. *Blood pressure of persons 18—74 years in the United States 1971—1972.* Rockville, Maryland: Public Health Service publication HRA 75-1632, 1975.
Roberts, J. *Hearing status and ear examination findings among adults.* Washington, D.C.: Public Health Service publication 1000, series 11, no. 32, 1968a.
Roberts, I. *Monocular-binocular visual acuity of adults.* Washington, D.C.: Public Health Service publication 1000, series 11, no. 30, 1968b.
Roberts, J. *Binocular visual acuity of adults by region and selected demographic characteristics.* Washington, D.C.: Public Health Service publication 1000, series 11, no. 25, 1967.
Roberts, J. *Weight by height and age of adults.* Washington, D.C.:

Public Health Service publication 1000, series 11, no. 14, 1966.
Roberts J. *Binocular visual acuity of adults.* Washington, D.C.: Public Health Service publication 1000, series, no. 3, 1964.
Roberts, J. and Bayliss, D. *Hearing levels of adults by race, region, and area of residence.* Washington, D.C.: Public Health Service publication 1000, series 11, no. 26, 1967.
Roberts, J. and Cohrssen, J. *Hearing levels of adults by education, income, and occupation.* Washington, D.C.: Public Health Service publication 1000, series 11, no. 31, 1968a.
Roberts, I. and Cohrssen, J. *History and examination findings related to visual acuity among adults.* Washington, D.C.: Public Health Service publication 1000, series 11, no. 28, 1968b.
Robinson, A.B. Why do we age? Can we diminish the rate and debilitating effect of aging? *Linus Pauling Institute Newsletter,* 1978, *1,* (June), 3.
Rockstein, M., Sussman, M., and Chesky,J. (Editors). *Theoretical aspects of aging.* New York: Academic Press, 1974.
Rodale, J.I. (Editor). *The encyclopedia of common diseases.* Emmaus, Pennsylvania: Rodale Books, Inc., 1973.
Rohte, 0. and Muntzing, J. Effects of reserpine, 6-hydroxydopamine, pchlorophenylalanine and a combination of these substances on the grooming behavior of mice. *Psychopharmacologia,* 1973, *31,* 333—342
Rose, C.L. *Measurement of social age. Aging and Human Development,* 1972, *3,* 153.
Rose, C.L. Social factors in longevity. *The Gerontologist,* 1964, 4, 27-37 Rose, C.L. and Bell, B. *Predicting longevity: methodology and critique.*
Lexington, Mass.: Heath, 1971.
Rose, C.L., Enslein, K. and Nuttall, R.L. Univariate and multivariate findings from a longevity study. *Proceedings of the 20th annual meeting of the Gerontological Society,* 1967, 42.
Rosee, B.G. Untersuchungen ueber das normale Hoervermoegen in den verschiedenen Lebensaltern unter besonderer Beruecksichtigung der Pruefung mit dem Audiometer. *Zeitsch rift fuer Laryngologie, Rhinologie, Otologie, und ihre Grenzgebiete,* 1953, *32,* 414—420.

Rosen, S., Plester, D., El-Mofty, E., and Rosen, H.V. High frequency audiometry in presbycusis; a comparative study of the Mabaan tribe in the Sudan with urban populations. *Archives of Otolaryngology,* 1964, 79, 18—32.

Rosenberg, B. *Personal communication,* October 31, 1975. Rosenberg, B. Kemeny, G., Smith, L.G., Skurnick, I.D., and Bandursky, M.J. The kinetics and thermodynamics of death in multi cellular organisms. *Mechanisms of Aging and Development,* 1973, *2,* 275—293.

Rosenberg, B., Kemeny, G., Switzer, R.C., and Hamilton, T.C. Quantitative evidence for protein denaturation as the cause of thermal death. *Nature,* 1971, *232,* 471.

Rosenfeld, A. *The second genesis.* Englewood Cliffs, New Jersey: Prentice-Hall, 1969.

Rosenthal, R. Experimenter expectancy and the reassuring nature of the null hypothesis decision procedure. *Psychological Bulletin,* 1968, *70,* 30—47.

Rosenthal, R. On the social psychology of the psychological experiment: the experimenter's hypothesis as an unintended determinant of experimental results. *American Scientist,* 1963, 268—283.

Ross, M.H. Length of life and nutrition in the rat. *Journal of Nutrition,* 1961, *75,* 197-210.

Ross, M.H. and Bras, G. Food preference and length of life. *Science,* 1975, *190,* October 10, 165—167.

Rozin, M.I. The physiological mechanism of the conditioned reflex to time. *Academy of Sciences Proceedings, Byelorussian SSR, 1959,3,* no. 7, July, 318—321.

Ruitenbeek, H.M. (Editor). *Going crazy: the radical therapy of R.D. Laing and others.* New York: Bantam, 1972.

Rush, B. *Medical inquiries and observations.* Philadelphia: J. Conrad, 1805. Ryzl, M. Training the psi faculty by hypnosis. *Journal of the Society of Psychic Research,* 1962, *41,* 234.

Sauer, H.I. and Parke, D.W. Counties with extreme death rates and associated factors. *American Journal of Epidemiology,* 1974, 99, 258-264.

Schaie, K.W. *Theory and methods of research on aging.* Morgantown, West Virginia: West Virginia University, 1968.
Schaie, K.W. and Gribbon, K. Adult development and aging. *Annual Review of Psychology,* 1975, *26,* 65—96.
Scheinfeld, A. Mortality of men and women. *Scientific American,* 1958, *198,* 22-27.
Schmeidler, G.R. Rorschach and ESP scores of patients suffering from cerebral concussion. *Journal of Parapsychology,* 1952, *16,* 80.
Schmeidler, G.R. Picture frustration ratings and ESP scores for subjects who showed moderate annoyance at the ESP task. *Journal of Parapsychology,* 1954, *18,* 137.
Schneck, J.M. Audiometry under hypnosis. *Psychosomatic Medicine,* 1948, *10,* 361—365.
Schneck, J.M. *Studies in scientific hypnosis.* New York: Nervous and Mental Disease Monographs, 1945.
Schneck, J.M. and Bergman, M. Auditory acuity for pure tones in the waking and hypnotic states. *Journal of Speech and Hearing Disorders.* 1949, *14,* 33-36.
Schrag, P. and Divoky, D. *The myth of the hyperactive child: and other means of child control,* New York: Pantheon, 1975.
Schultz, J.H. *Das autogene training.* Stuttgart: Georg Thieme Verlag, 1932.
Schultz, J.H. and Luthe, W. *Autogenic training.* New York: Grune & Stratton, 1959.
Schwartz, G.E. Voluntary control of human cardiovascular integration and differentiation through feedback and reward. *Science,* 1972, *175,* No. 4017, 90—93.
Schwartz, Len. *The World of the Unborn: Nurturing your Child before Birth.* New York: Marek, 1980.
Scogin, F.; Prohaska, M. *Aiding Older Adults with Memory Complaints.* Sarasota, Flordia, Professional Resource Exchange, 1993, Pb.
Scott, J.P., Lee, C.T., Ho, J.E. Effects of fighting, genotype, and amphetamine sulfate on body temperature of mice. *Journal of Comparative and Physiological Psychology,* 1971, 76, 349—352.

Bibliography

Scott, J.P., and Marston, M.V. Non-adaptive behavior resulting from a series of defeats in githing mice. *Journal of Abnormal and Social Psychology,* 1953, *48,* 417—428.

Segerberg, 0. *The immortality factor.* New York: Dutton, 1974.

Selye, H. *Stress without distress.* New York: Signet, 1975.

Sheehy, Gail. *New Passages.* New York, Ballantine Books (Trd Pap), 1996.

Shock, N.W. The physiology of aging. *Scientific American,* 1962, *206,* 100-110.

Shock, N.W. Physiological aspects of mental disorders in later life. In O. Kaplan (Editor) *Mental disorders in later life.* Stanford: Stanford University Press, 1945, Ch. 3.

Shock, N.W. Classified bibliography of gerontology and geriatrics Stanford: Stanford University Press, 1951. Also: monthly up dates since 1951 in the *Journal of Gerontology.*

Shor, R.E. and Orne, E.C. Norms on the Harvard Group Scale of Hypnotic Susceptibility, Form A. *international Journal of Clinical and Experimental Hypnosis,* 1963, *11,* 39—47.

Shor, R.E. and Orne, E.C. *Harvard Group Scale of Hypnotic Susceptibility, Form A.* Palo Alto: Consulting Psychologists Press, 1962.

Silberberg, R., Jarett, S.R., and Silberberg, M. Longevity of female mice kept on various dietary regimens during growth. *Journal of Gerontology,* 1962, *17,* 239—255.

Silberberg, M. and Silberberg, R. Diet and life span. *Physiological Review, 1955, 35,* 347-362.

Simmons, D. Experiments on the alleged sharpening of razor blades and the preservation of flowers by pyramids. *New Horizons,* 1973, Summer.

Simonton, C., Simonton, S., and Creighton, J. *Getting well again.* Los Angeles: J.P. Tarcher, 1978.

Sinclair, D. *Human growth after birth, second edition.* London: Oxford University Press, 1973.

Siroka, R.W., Siroka, E.K., and Schloss, G.A. *Sensitivitytrainingand group encounter.* New York: Grosset & Dunlap, 1971.

Smith, W.H. The effects of hypnosis and suggestion upon auditory threshold. *Journal of Speech and Hearing Research,* 1969, 12,161—168.

Spoor, A. Presbycusis values in relation to noise induced hearing loss. *International audiology,* 1967, 6, 48—57.
Stamler, J. and Epstein, F.M. Coronary heart disease: risk factors as guides to preventive action. *Preventive Medicine,* 1972, *1,* 27—48.
Steinhaus, H. Untersuchungen ueber den Zusammenhang von Presbyopie und Lebensdauer, unter Beruecksichtigungen der Todesursachen. *Archiven fuer Augenkunde,* 1932, *105,* 731—760.
Sterling, K. and Miller, J.G. The effects of hypnosis upon visual and auditory acuity. *American Journal of Psychology,* 1940, *53,* 269—276.
Sternglass, E.J. *Low-level radiation.* New York: Ballantine, 1972.
Stewart, K. Dream theory in Malaya. In C.T. Tart (Editor) *A Itered states of consciousness.* New York: Wiley, 1969, Ch. 9, 159—167.
Still, H. *Of time, tides, and inner clocks.* Moonachie, New Jersey: Pyramid Publications, 1972.
Stoller, E.P.; Gibson, R.C. *Worlds of Difference: Inequity in the Aging Experience, 2nd edition.* Thousand Oaks, CA, Pine Forge Press, 1997.
Storandt, M.; Vandenbos, G.R. editor. *The Adult Years: Continuity and Change.* Washington, D.C., APA 1989.
Stoudt, H.W., Damon, A., McFarland, R.A. and Roberts J. *Skinfolds, body girths, biacromial diameter, and selected anthropometric indices of adults.* Washington, D.C.: Public Health Service publication 1000, series 11, no. 35, 1970.
Strebler, B.L. Genetic and cellular aspects of life span prediction. In Palmore, E. and Jeffers, F. (Editors) *Prediction of lifespan.* Lexington, Mass.: Heath, 1971, 33—49.
Strehler, B.L. *Time, cells, and aging.* New York: Academic Press, 1962. Strehler, B.L. Studies on the comparative physiology of aging. II. On the mechanism of temperature life shortening in Drosophila melanogaster. *Journal of Gerontology,* 1961, *16,* 2.
Strosberg, I.M. and Vic, I. I. Physiologic changes in the eye during hypnosis. *American Journal of Clinical Hypnosis,* 1962, 4, 242—267.

Bibliography

Stuart, Friend (Stuart Otto). *How to conquer physical death.* San Marcos, California: Dominion Press, 1968.

Stuchlikova, E., Juricova-Horakova, M., and Deyl, Z. New aspects of the dietary effect of life prolongation in rodents; what is the role of obesity in aging? *Experimental Gerontology,* 1975, *10,* 141—144.

Sturgeon, P., Beller, S., and Bates, E. Study of blood group factors in longevity. *Journal of Gerontology,* 1969, *24,* 90—94.

Swenson, W.M. Attitudes toward death among the aged. In Fulton, R. (Editor) *Death and identity.* New York: Wiley, 1965.

Tait, E.F. Accommodative convergence. *American Journal of Ophthalmology,* 1951, *34,* 1093—1107.

Tannenbaum. A. Effects of varying caloric intake upon tumor incidence and tumor growth. *Annals of the New York Academy of Science,* 1947, 49, 5-18.

Tappel, A.L. Will anti-oxidant nutrients slow aging process? *Geriatrics,* 1968, *23,* 97-105.

Tart, C.T. (Editor). *Altered states of consciousness: a book of readings.* New York: Wiley, 1969.

Taub, H.A. Visual short-term memory as a function of age, rate of presentation, and schedule of presentation. *Journal of Gerontology* 1966, *21,* 388—391.

Ten Ham, M. and de Jong, Y. Absence of interaction between D9-tetrahydrocannabinol (D9-THC) and cannabidol (CBD) in aggression, muscle control, and body temperature experiments in mice. *Psycho-pharmacologia,* 1975, *41,* 169—174.

Ten Ham, M. and de Jong, Y. Tolerance to the hypothermic and aggression-attenuating effects of D—8 and D-9 tetrahydrocannabinol in mice. *European Journal of Pharmacology,* 1974, *28,* 144—148.

Thomson, G. *The foreseeable future.* Cambridge, England: University Press, 1955.

Tibbitts, C. and Donahue, W. (Editors). *Social and psychological aspects of aging: aging around the world: Proceedings of the Fifth Congress of the International Association of Gerontology in San Francisco, 1960.*

Timiras, P.S. *Developmental physiology and aging.* New York: Macmillan, 1972.
Toms, M. Birth without violence: interview with Dr. Frederick LeBoyer. *New Age Journal,* 1975, 1(8), October, 14—21.
Tong, B.R. The ghetto of the mind: notes on the historical psychology of Chinese America. *AmerAsia Journal,* 1971, *1(3),* 1—31.
Toomin, M.K. and Toomin, H. Biofeedback—fact and fantasy: does it hold implication for gifted education? *Gifted Child Quarterly,* 1973, *17,* 48—55.
Toth, M. and Neilson, G. *Pyramid power.* New York: Freeway Press, 1974.
Travis, L.E. Suggestibility and negativism as measured by the auditory threshold during reverie. *Journal of Abnormal Psychology.* 1924, *18,* 351—382.
Treloar, W.W. Review of recent research on hypnotic learning. *Psychological Reports,* 1967, *20,* 723—732.
Trimmer, E.J. *Rejuvenation.* New York: Barnes, 1970.
Tryon, R.C. Genetic differences in maze-learning ability in rats. *Yearbook of the National Society of Studies in Education,* 1940, *39,* 111—119.
Veiny, Thomas. *The Secret Life of the Unborn Child.* New York: Simon & Schuster, 1981.
Vishnudevananda, S. *The complete illustrated book of yoga.* New York: Bell, 1960.
Von Lerchenthal, P. Death from psychic causes. *Bulletin of the Menninger Clinic,* 1948, *12,* 31—36.
Von Uexkull, J. A stroll through the worlds of animals and men. In C.H. Schiller (Editor) *Instinctive behavior.* New York: International Universities Press, 1957, 5—80.
Wade, C. *The rejuvenation vitamin.* New York: Award Books, 1970.
Wade, N. Recombinant DNA: NIH sets strict rules to launch new technology. *Science,* 1975, *190,* no. 4220, December 19, 1175—1179.
Walk, D.E. Finger dexterity of the pressure suited subject on the Purdue Pegboard Dexterity Test. *United States Air Force AMRC-TDR* no. 64-41, *1965.*

Bibliography

Wallace, R.K., Jacobs, D.E., and Harnington, B. Reversal of biological aging in subjects practising the transcendental meditation technique. Paper delivered to the 36th annual meeting of the American Geriatrics Society, April, 1979.

Walters, M.H. Psychic death: report of a possible case. *Archives of neurology and psychiatry,* 1944, *52,* 84—85.

Warner, S.J. *Self-realization and self-defeat.* New York: Grove Press, 1966.

Watson, L. *Supernature.* New York: Doubleday, 1973.

Weale, R.A. The eye and measurement of aging rate. *Lancet,* 1970, 1, 147.

Weitz, C.A. The effects of aging and habitual activity pattern on exercise performance among a high altitude Nepalese population. *Dissertation Abstracts International,* 1974, *35,* 1303A (University Microfilms 74—20,978). Doctoral dissertation completed at Pennsylvania State University.

Weitzenhoffer, A.M. Explorations in hypnotic time distortions. I. Acquisitions of temporal reference frames under conditions of time distortion. *Journal of Nervous and Mental Diseases,* 1964, *138,* 354. Weitzenhoffer, A.M. *General techniques of hypnotism.* New York: Grune & Stratton, 1957.

Weitzenhoffer, A.M. *Hypnotism: an objective study in suggestibility.* New York: Wiley, 1953.

Welch, L. The space and time of induced hypnotic dreams. *Journal of Psychology,* 1935, *1,* 171—178.

Welford, A.T. Experimental psychology in the study of aging. *British Medical Bulletin.* 1964, *20,* 65—69.

Welford, A.T. Changes of performance time with age: a correction and methodological note. *Ergonomics,* 1962, *5,* 581—582.

Welford, A.T. *Aging and human skill.* London: Oxford University Press, 1958.

Welford, A.T. and Birren, J.E. (Editors). *Behaviour, aging, and the nervous system: biological determinants of speed of behaviour and its changes with age.* Springfield, Illinois: Thomas, 1965.

Wells, W.R. Expectancy versus performance in hypnosis. *Journal of General Psychology,* 1946, *35,* 99—119.

Westra, A. and Dewey, W.C. Variation in sensitivity to heat shock during the cell-cycle of Chinese hamster cells in vitro. *Interna-*

tional Journal of Radiation Biology, 1971, *19,* 467.
Whitbourne, S.K. *The Aging Individual: Physical & Psychological Perspectives.* New York., Springer Publishing Co., 1996.
White, J. *Everything you want to know about TM.* New York: Pocket Books, 1976.
White, R.W. *The abnormal personality.* New York: Ronald, 1956,504—510. And all subsequent editions to the present.
Wiesner, B.P. and Sheard, N.M. The duration of life in an albino rat population. *Proceedings of the Royal Society (Edinburgh),* 1934, *55,* 1.
Williams, P., Tibbitts, C. and Donahue, W. (Editors). *Processes of aging: I.* New York: Atherton, 1963, 184—197.
Williams, R.J. *Nutrition against disease.* New York: Pitman, 1973.
Wit, A. and Wang, S.C. Temperature-sensitive neurons in preopticlantenor hypothalamic region: actions of pyrogen and acetylsalicylate. *American Journal of Physiology,* 1968, *215,* 1160—1169.
Witte, N.K., Kryshanowskaja, W.W., and Steshenskaya, E.I. The process of aging in the light of work physiology. *Zeitschrift fur Altersforschung,* 1967, *20,* 91—98.
Wohlwill, J.F. The age variable in psychological research. *Psychological Review,* 1970, 77, 49—64.
Wolman, B.B. (Editor). *Handbook of general psychology.* Englewood Cliffs, New Jersey: Prentice-Hall, 1973.
Wolstenholmes, G.E.W. and O'Connor, M. (Editors). *The lifespan of animals.* Boston: Little, Brown & Co., 1959.
Woodrow, H. Time perception. In S.S. Stevens (Editor). *Handbook of experimental psychology,* New York: Wiley, 1951.
Woodruff, D.S. Relationships between EEG alpha frequency, reaction, time, and age; a biofeedback study. *Psychophysiology,* 1975, *12,* 673-681. From the doctoral dissertation, University of Southern California, 1972.
Woodruff, D. and Birren, J.E. (Editors). *Aging: scientific perspectives and social issues.* New York: D. Van Nostrand, 1975.
World Health Organization. *World Health Statistics Annual, 1971, volume 1: Vital statistics and causes of death.* Geneva: World Health Organization, 1974.

Bibliography

Yacorzynski, G.K. Organic mental disorders. In B.B. Wolman (Editor) *Handbook of clinical psychology.* New York: McGraw-Hill, 1965, 362-365.

Yagiela, I.A., McCarthy, D.D., Gibb, J.W. The effect of hypothermic doses of 1-D9-tetrahydrocannabinol on biogenic amine metabolism in selected parts of the rat brain. *Life Sciences,* 1974, *14,* 2367-2378.

Yogananda, P. *Metaphysical meditations.* Los Angeles: Self-Realization Fellowship, 1964.

Yogi, M.M. *Transcendental meditation.* New York: Signet, 1968.

Yuan, G.C. and Chang, R.S. Testing of compounds for capacity to prolong post-mitotic life span of cultured human amion cells: effects of steroids and Panax ginseng. *Journal of Gerontology,* 1969, *24,* 82-85.

Zarit, S.; Knight, B.G., editors. *A Guide to Psychotherpy & Aging: Effective Clinical Interventions in a Life State Context.* Washington, D.C., APA, 1998

Zimbardo, P.G., Marshall, G., and Maslach, C. Liberating behavior from time-bound control: expanding the present through hypnosis. *Journal of Applied Social Psychology,* 1971, *1,* 305—323.

Zimbardo, P.G. The human choice: individuation, reason, and order versus deindividuation, impulse, and chaos. In W.J. Arnold and D. Levine (Editors) *Nebraska symposium on motivation.* Lincoln, Nebraska: University of Nebraska Press, 1969.

Growing Younger

The Adult Growth Examination

TEST MANUAL

Note:

THE ADULT GROWTH EXAMINATION manual is reproduced here in its entirety. In order to allow for its use as a complete handbook independent of the main text, certain sections and some of the charts appear in the book as well as in the manual.

CONTENTS

Part 1. Directions for Administration and Scoring 219
    Test Materials 219
    Time Requirements 220
    Administering the Test 220
    Test Procedure 221
    Scoring the Test 224
    Interpreting the Test 224
    Sample AGE score sheet 226
    Sample AGE monitor record 227

    Body Age Tables:
    1. Decade Chart of Aging for Men 228
    2. Decade Chart of Aging for Women 229
    3. Conversion: Hearing Loss (HL) to Body Age 229
    4. Conversion: Near Vision (NPV) to Body Age 232
    5. Conversion: Systolic Blood Pressure (SBP) to Body Age 234
    6. Expected Relationship between Birth Age and Body Age 237

Part 2. General Test Information and Background 239
    Test Construction 242
    Test Standardization 243
    Establishment of Norms 243
    Reliability 244
    Validity 244
    Uses 245

    Reprinted Tables:
    7. & 8. Reliability 250
    9. & 10. Validity 251-252
    11. & 12. Comparative Uses 253-254

Bibliography 255

Part I

DIRECTIONS FOR ADMINISTRATION AND SCORING

You DO NOT have to be a psychologist or a physician to give the *Adult Growth Examination* (AGE). On the other hand, you may wish to consult such professionals to interpret any results significantly different from the calendar age. What you do need to give this test effectively is a practiced familiarity with the test materials and careful adherence to the instructions. Courses in psychological testing, assessment of adult aging and gerontology would also be helpful. After sufficient supervised practice, the AGE may be used by any intelligent adults to monitor their body age and the relative aging of friends and family. The test may also be used professionally by psychologists, physicians, mental health workers, nurses, researchers and other specialists in the health or life sciences.

Test Materials
A complete test kit will include a manual, a portable electronic blood pressure monitor, a portable audiometric monitor, a portable visual near-point indicator and visual target cards. A pack of score sheets and a carrying case for the equipment will also be required.

Portable electronic blood pressure monitor: Battery operated, with solid-state circuitry. Allows accurate rapid measurement without a stethoscope. Cuff microphone, red signal light on instrument panel, monitor panel of at least 2.5" with at least one marked division for every 2 mm/hg.

Growing Younger

Portable audiometric monitor: Operates on normal AC wall current. Solid-state circuitry, stereo earphones, microphone, variable volume dial (up to 59 dbs by increments of 1 db), two frequencies of 1000 cps and 6000 cps. Hearing level tested.

Portable visual near point indicator: Visual target cards with pica type sentence (3 different sentences for 3 different cards), card insert on graded measurement ruler expandable up to 65 inches. Near point of clear focus tested.

Score sheets.

Time Requirements
Most people can be tested in ten to fifteen minutes on this untimed test. Relaxed accuracy is much more important than speed.

Administering the Test
General Suggestions:
1. Set up the test equipment in a quiet, well-illuminated room with ample room to move.
2. The examiner should be relaxed, positive and. encouraging. Postpone irrelevant discussion until all measurements have been completed. Discussion of the test's background, meaning or purpose should not be done during the actual testing.
3. Directions to the person being examined should be read aloud rather than given from memory. It is useful to have the persons being examined follow the reading of the directions on their own copy.
4. Never rush the person being examined.
5. It is often useful to give the test several times to the same person, perhaps a few days apart and at varying hours. This will determine the individual stability or reliability of the body age score.
6. Significantly high or unusual age results should be referred to a health professional. Persons tested should be told that this test, like all tests, is subject to error. Results should be carefully double-checked before any serious personal or research decisions are made in consequence. The most frequent use of the test will be for personal knowledge. As such, it can lead to a greater enjoyment of life if properly used.

The Adult Growth Examination

7. Before administering the test, individuals should know its purpose and provide their clear consent. In addition, the examinee must be given the results at the end of the test in a clear and comprehensive form. Since confidentiality has been promised, it must be honored. Also, no test result is irreversible.
8. Professional standards of ethics and law for human testing or research apply to this test.

Test Procedure

A. The person to be tested (the examinee) is seated on a comfortable chair next to a table. On the table is the score sheet, which then is completed to provide basic background information.

B. The examiner reads: *"You are about to have a short, painless series of tests of health measures associated with aging. You may let the examiner know when the directions are not clear but otherwise please hold all questions until the test series is over. Do I have your consent to begin?"*

C. With consent, the first blood pressure measurement is made. The examiner reads: *"This will be the first of three blood pressure readings to be taken in the test series."* The blood pressure measurement is made with the subject wearing the blood pressure monitor cuff over the bulge in the upper left arm. This places the cuff microphone directly over the brachial artery. The cuff is then plugged into the instrument case, the instrument is switched on and the air valve is closed by rotating the cap clockwise with the thumb and forefinger. The cuff is then inflated by pumping the hand bulb. The light may flash on the control panel while the cuff is moved or inflated; this is caused by noise picked up by the sensitive microphone in the cuff. The red flashing will cease when the inflation has stopped and pressure is above systolic pressure (inflate to about the systolic pressure you would expect at 20 calendar years above the age of the person being tested, up to a maximum pressure of 160 mm/hg). The cuff is then *slowly* deflated by gradually opening the air valve and turning the cap counterclockwise. The first flash on the dial occurs at systolic pressure (the maximum pressure in the arteries when heart is not at rest) and the pressure must be read at exactly that in-

Growing Younger

stant. When the reading has been made, let out all the pressure. Leave the cuff loose and uninflated on the left arm. Record the first systolic blood pressure reading on the score sheet. (Note: Corday & Vyden, 1966, have shown that blood pressure will go up 10-30 mmlhg up to 45 minutes after eating; they also found that excessively warm surroundings lowered blood pressure while excessively cold surroundings raised it. It therefore makes sense to test only in a comfortably temperate room and not after the examinee has just finished eating.)

D. On to the hearing test. The examiner reads: *"Next is a hearing test. Please put on the earphones. Make sure they are firmly on your ears but are not so tight as to be painful."* When this is done, the examiner speaks through the portable audiometric monitor's (PAM) microphone and continues: *"Nod if you can hear me. All right. Now I would like you to turn so that your back is to me. This will help you concentrate on the sound in the earphones without the distraction of seeing the tones turned on. It also helps me keep from letting you know when I am sounding a tone."* Tune PAM to 1000 cps at 40 db for the right ear. *"When you hear a tone in your right ear, raise your right hand all the way up ... like this"* (sound tone). *"When you hear a tone in your left ear, raise your left hand all the way up . . . like this"* (switch to left ear and sound tone). *"Good. Be sure to raise your hand all the way up on the side you hear the tone when you can hear the tone. We are now ready to start the test."* The frequency is still set at 1000 cps. This is a normal conversation frequency and is not an age measure. It is used to warm up the examinee to the test and to get a rough indication of the quality of normal hearing. It is also a chance to make sure the equipment is in good order. Test first the right ear and then the left. Use one-second tones. Begin testing each ear at 50 dbs. If no hand goes up at that level, raise up to 59. If at 59 db, the hand has still not gone up, cut in with the microphone and reread the directions. If still no success, check PAM and see if the examinee has fallen asleep. Most people will raise their arm at 50 db. If so, decrease the volume by gradual steps until you find the volume level so low that the examinee hears it only about half the time. Record that as the hearing level score for each ear. Now do the same for each ear at the age-related high frequency of 6000 cps. The

The Adult Growth Examination

"better ear" score is the lowest volume in db scored at 6000 cps, whether it is the right or the left ear. Turn off PAM.

E. Time for another blood pressure test. After removing the earphones, the examinee turns in the chair to again face the examiner. When comfortable, the examinee is told: *"This is the second of three blood pressure readings to be taken in this series."* Inflate the cuff to about 20 mm/hg higher than the first systolic reading (up to 160 maximum). Take and record the second systolic blood pressure reading. Then, leaving the cuff loose on the left arm, go on to the vision test.

F. The examiner reads: *"This is a test of near vision or how closely you can see printed material without any blurring."* One of the three target cards is inserted in the near point indicator (NP!) at the far end from the examinee. Lighting should be excellent and without glare. *"Look down the ruler to the far end, where you see a white card. lam going to move this card toward you until you can see the printed letters on it clearly. Say when. Good. Now lam going to keep moving it toward you very slowly. Tell me when it begins to blur in any way. All right. Now I am going to move the card away from you. Tell me when it stops blurring."* In this manner, the distance at which the sentence on the card blurs is recorded. No glasses are allowed. Record distance to the nearest tenth of an inch if at all possible. Any one of the three target cards may be used; alternatives are for retesting. When done, the examinee is again made comfortable in the chair.

G. The examiner reads: *"This is the third of three blood pressure readings to be taken in this test series."* Again inflate the cuff to about 20 mm/hg higher than the last reading (up to 160 maximum). Take and record the third systolic blood pressure reading. Then, remove the cuff from the examinee's arm and turn off the machine. Make sure all equipment is off. Compute the average of the three systolic blood pressure readings and record that on the score sheet. Thank the examinee for the time and cooperation. Set an appointment for a later date to present and explain the results, once they are determined by converting raw scores to body age scores.

Scoring the Test

Using the conversion tables (which follow), convert the raw score for each subtest into the equivalent age score. Then rank order the three scores. The middle one or median (neither the highest nor the lowest) is the tested body age of the examinee. It is your best estimate of the body age at the time of testing. Additional measures, listed in the decade charts following in this manual, may be used as supplementary indicators of aging if available from professional medical, dental or psychological testing. If for any reason you have been unable to use one of the three basic subtests, average the two body age scores you have measured as the best estimate available of bodily aging (e.g., as with a blind or deaf examinee).

Interpreting the Test

⇒ Read the entire manual before interpreting body age scores.

⇒ No test score is the final word. Even if completely accurate, there are always many ways to improve it for better or for worse.

⇒ The body age scale goes from 19 to 71 years. Those with body ages under 19 or over 71 will be off the scale and not precisely assessed. As such, the test is most likely to capture exact body ages for the 30 to 60 calendar-age set. Until norms for older people are available, it will not be useful for those over 70 unless they are very youthful for their age.

⇒ There is a little fluctuation in body age from one test to the next. However, an age score that is consistently at least *10 years* above or below the calendar age may be viewed as significantly older or younger in body age than the generation born the same year (two standard deviations away).

⇒ In addition to the overall body age score, if a subtest score is 10 or more years beyond what your calendar age indicates it should be, a confirming visit to a relevant medical specialist is indicated. With systolic blood pressure raw scores, 140 mm/hg is borderline hypertension and 160 mm/hg (at any age) is definite hypertension (Gordon & Devine, 1966). The American Heart Association (1975) considers normal systolic blood pressure to be under 120 mm/hg; over 150 mm/hg the heart attack risk has doubled and the stroke risk has quadrupled. The AHA also de-

The Adult Growth Examination

fines a normal cholesterol level as below 194 mg.% with any excess of 250 mg.% tripling the risk of heart attack or stroke.

⇒ Those who are involved in reversing the aging processes generally choose 19-year subtest levels as their objective.

⇒ As with any test, the norms will need regular updating and expansion. It is meant primarily for your information, enjoyment and self awareness. It is a test of aging and as such is no substitute for a comprehensive health examination.

On the next page is a sample score sheet. Following that are two decade charts of the basic three subtests and five supplementary measures of aging. Next are the conversion tables for determining body age from raw test scores.

Growing Younger

Adult Growth Examination
Score Sheet

Name _____ Date of Birth _____
Identifying Number _____
Address _____
Telephone _____ Sex _____
Occupation _____ Education _____
Marital Status _____ Referred by _____
Medical Problems _____

I know the purpose of this test and consent to take it of my own free will. I understand the results will be handled in a professional and ethical manner.

_____
Signature and Date

The Examiner: _____

Time test begun _____

Measurements   Body Temperature _____
SBP-1 Systolic blood pressure _____ mm/hg
HL Hearing loss at 1000 cps: Right ear _____ db Left ear _____ db
HL Hearing loss at 6000 cps: Right ear _____ db Left ear _____ db
HL Hearing loss at 6000 cps: Better ear _____ db*
SBP-2 Systolic blood pressure _____ mm/hg
NPV Near point vision _____ inches*
SBP-3 Systolic blood pressure _____ mm/hg
SBP Average of three readings _____ mm/hg*
Time test concluded _____ Total testing time _____ minutes

Results
*HL raw score _____ HL age score _____ BODY AGE _____
*NPV raw score _____ NPV age score _____ BIRTH AGE ____
*SBP raw score _____ SBP age score _____ Difference _____

The Adult Growth Examination

Adult Growth Examination
Monitor Record

Name _____

Date of Testing	Body Age:	NPV	SBP	HL	Total	Birth Age	Difference

Every other space may be left to record intervening activity.

Growing Younger

Body Age Tables

Table 1. Decade Chart of Aging for Men
Three Basic Measures & Five Supplementary Measures

Measure	20+	30+	40+	50+	60+	70+	Units
Basic							
Hearing HL	+4	+12	+17	+22	+38	+52	Decibels
Vision NPV	4.0	5.5	9.0	15.0	39.0	63.0	inches
Blood SBP	121	125	129	134	144	149	Mm/Hg. %
Supplementary:							
Dexterity FD	48	47	45	42	37	34	filled holes 4 min.
Glucose GT	95	102	115	118	130	140	mg. %
Cholesterol CL	178	206	227	231	233	- - - *	mg. %
Peridontal PI	0.62	0.92	1.27	1.62	2.15	2.50	peridontal index
Tooth Decay DMF	14	16	18	21	24	27	No. teeth DMF

*no further increase with age.

Note: These norms and the procedures used to derive them may be found in their original sources as follows:

HL: Glorig & Roberts, 1965; Roberts, 1968b; Morgan, 1966-1972. Cf Corson, 1959; Rosen et a!., 1964; Spoor, 1967

NPV: Chapanis, 1949, 1956; Roberts 1964-68; Morgan, 1966-72. Cf Heidemann, 1932; Steinhaus, 1932; Bernstein, 1945; Friedenwald, 1952; Bruckner, 1959

SBP: Gordon, 1964; Morgan, 1966-72. Cf. Roberts, *1975.*

FD: Walk, 1965; Gavurin, 1963; Morgan, 1971.

CT: Garst, 1966; Florey, 1969; Morgan, 196gb, 1971.

CL: Moore, 1967; Florey, 1969; Morgan, 196gb, 1971.

Pl: Kelly, 1965; Morgan, 1968b, 1971; Johnson *et al.,* 1965.

DMF: Kelly, 1967; Morgan, 196gb, 1971; Johnson *et al.,* 1965.

See bibliography at end of text for complete citations.

The Adult Growth Examination

Table 2. Decade Chart of Aging for Women
Three Basic Measures & Five Supplementary Measures

Measure	20+	30+	40+	50+	60+	70+	Units
Basic							
Hearing HL	+0	+5	+8	+12	+21	+27	Decibels
Vision NPV	4.0	5.5	9.0	15.0	39.0	63.0	inches
Blood SBP	111	116	123	134	142	160	Mm/Hg. %
Supplementary:							
Dexterity FD	48	47	45	42	37	34	filled holes 4 min.
Glucose GT	104	110	118	133	145	160	mg. %
Cholesterol CL	185	198	214	237	262	266	mg. %
Peridontal PI	0.48	0.60	1.82	1.23	2.56	1.62	peridontal index
Tooth Decay DMF	14	18	20	22	26	28	no. teeth DMF

Note: These norms and the procedures used to derive them may be found in their original sources listed below Table 1 on the preceding page. The conversion tables of the next three pages also derive from primary sources as listed by subject measure below Table 1 on the preceding page.

Table 3 Conversion Table—Hearing Loss HL
Raw Scores to Body Age Scores

Hearing Loss HL in decibles	Men: Body Age in years	Women: Body Age in years
0	19-	20
1	19-	23
2	19-	25
3	19-	27

Growing Younger

Hearing Loss HL in decibles	Men: Body Age in years	Women: Body Age in years
4	20	29
5	21	32
6	22	35
7	24	39
8	25	41
9	27	44
10	28	45
11	29	48
12	31	50
13	34	51
14	35	52
15	38	53
16	39	54
17	41	56
18	43	58
19	45	58
20	46	59
21	48	60
22	50	61
23	50	63
24	51	65
25	52	66
26	52	68
27	53	70

The Adult Growth Examination

Hearing Loss HL in decibles	Men: Body Age in years	Women: Body Age in years
28	54	71+
29	54	71+
30	55	71+
31	55	71+
32	56	71+
33	57	71+
34	57	71+
35	58	71+
36-37	59	71+
38	60	71+
39-40	61	71+
41	62	71+
42-43	63	71+
44	64	71+
45	65	71+
46-47	66	71+
48	67	71+
49-50	68	71+
51	69	71+
52	70	71+
53+	71+	71+

Growing Younger

Table 4 Near Vision NPV
Raw Scores to Body Age Scores

Near Vision NPV in inches	Men and Women: Body Age in years
0.0-3.9	19-
4.0-4.1	20
4.2	21
4.3	22
4.4-4.5	23
4.6-4.7	24
4.8	25
4.9-5.0	26
5.1	27
5.2-5.3	28
5.4	29
5.5-5.7	30
5.8-6.1	31
6.2-6.5	32
6.6-6.8	33
6.9-7.1	34
7.2-7.5	35
7.6-7.9	36
8.0-8.2	37
8.3-8.5	38

The Adult Growth Examination

Near Vision NPV in inches	Men and Women: Body Age in years
8.6-8.9	39
9.0-9.5	40
9.6-10.1	41
10.2-10.7	42
10.8-11.3	43
11.4-11.9	44
12.0-12.5	45
12.6-13.1	46
13.2-13.7	47
13.8-14.3	48
14.4-14.9	49
15.0-17.3	50
17.4-19.7	51
19.8-22.1	52
22.2-24.5	53
24.6-26.9	54
27.0-29.3	55
29.4-31.7	56
31.8-34.1	57
34.2-36.5	58
36.6-38.9	59
39.0-41.3	60
41.4-43.7	61
43.8-46.1	62

Near Vision NPV in inches	Men and Women: Body Age in years
46.2-48.5	63
48.6-50.9	64
51.0-53.3	65
53.4-55.7	66
55.8-58.1	67
58.2-60.5	68
60.6-62.9	69
63.0-65.3	70
65.3+	71+

Table 5 Conversion Table: Systolic Blood Pressure SBP Raw Scores to Body Age Scores

Systolic Blood Pressure SBP mm. Hg. %	Men: Body Age in years	Women: Body Age in Years
0-110	19-	19-
111	19-	20
112	19-	21
113	19-	23
114	19-	25
115	19-	28
116	19-	30
117	19-	32
118	19-	33
119	19-	35

The Adult Growth Examination

Systolic Blood Pressure SBP mm. Hg. %	Men: Body Age in years	Women: Body Age in Years
120	19-	36
121	20	37
122	21	39
123	24	40
124	27	41
125	30	42
126	32	43
127	35	44
128	38	45
129	40	46
130	42	46
131	44	47
132	46	48
133	48	49
134	50	50
135	51	52
136	52	53
137	53	55
138	54	56
139	55	58
140	56	59
141	57	59
142	58	61
143	59	61

Growing Younger

Systolic Blood Pressure SBP mm. Hg. %	Men: Body Age in years	Women: Body Age in Years
144	60	62
145	63	62
146	65	63
147	67	63
148	69	64
149	71	64
150	72	65
151	73	65
152	74	66
153	76	66
154	77	67
155	78+	67
156-57	78+	68
158-59	78+	69
160	78+	70
161	78+	71+

Table 6   Expected Relationship Between Birth Age and Body Age

1. Birth age the same as body age: about 7% (1 in every 14) of those tested.

2. Birth age within ten years of body age: about 67% (2 of every 3) of those tested.

3. Birth age within five years of body age: about 47% (1 of every 2) of those tested.

4. Body age more than ten years *older* than birth age: about 16½% (1 of every 6) of those tested.

5. Body age more than ten years younger than birth age: about 16½% (1 of every 6) of those tested.

Note: From Morgan, 1994

Growing Younger

Part 2
GENERAL INFORMATION AND BACKGROUND

IT STARTED with Helmholtz. More than a century ago, in 1856, he wrote a handbook on the physiology of optics, which included the observation that there are individual differences in the optical physiology of aging. His specific focus was on "presbyopia" or the difficulty of seeing things clearly at close range, which is experienced by most people. Helmholtz noted that "persons with early progressing presbyopia die early and persons with late progressing presbyopia die late" (Bernstein, 1945, p. 378). Several decades later, the grand champion of individual differences (and the philosophical precursor of clinical psychology) Sir Francis Galton confirmed, after systematically testing more than 9,000 people aged 5 to 80 years, that both vision and hearing deteriorate with age (Galton, 1907).

Following up on the early work of Helmholtz and Galton, Steinhaus and his doctoral student Heidemann began a careful combing of 5,000 patients who had had eye difficulties over a long period of time. They published their results in 1932 in both dissertation and journal form. Although their sample was much narrower than Galton's 1884 survey, they did confirm, based on 1,000 death records, the very high correlation between presbyopia and mortality. In their sample they found presbyopia to be primarily a predictor of death by heart disease. They found presbyopia to be so potent an aging characteristic that it was unaffected in its progress by social class, rural/urban living, or sex differences. In 1945, mathematician Felix Bernstein suggested that these studies justified the use of presbyopia as the basis for an index of physiological aging.

It was an intelligent and well documented recommendation. It was also ignored by the scientific community. Nor did Bernstein go on to standardize a test based on his insight.

In 1949, a test of body age based on sexual functions was recommended by Benjamin. In 1951, Murray suggested a more practical approach based on vision, strength and other indices. He predicted body age would be as important a concept to the last half of the twentieth century as mental age was to the first. He recommended that insurance companies take a close look at this approach. They did not. Benjamin and Murray were not heard from again on this subject.

Also in 1951, H.B. Jones and colleagues promoted the "Lipo-Protein Index" as an index of aging. A basic blood test technique, it has often since been used to assess the risk of vascular disease. While the "Lipo-Protein Index" is a little too gross an index to yield year-by-year body age scores, it was still a step forward in that it called attention to the circulatory system as another fruitful direction for assessing body age. As we have seen, vision had been noticed by Helmholtz in 1856 and hearing by Galton in 1884. *(Cf.* Lipo-Protein Index in Birren, 1959, p. 352.)

In 1959, James Birren edited what is still one of the finest handbooks of aging extant: the *Handbook of Aging and the Individual: Psychological and Biological Aspects.* Birren called for the recognition of "functional age" since individuals age at.different rates. Again, body age was compared conceptually to mental age as an age-specific variable worth noting. For the next fifteen years, a number of distinguished gerontologists would call for a test of functional age, but without following through to standardize one themselves (and without giving Birren or his predecessors credit).

In 1960, Burgess presented a valuable interdisciplinary collection of objective measures of aging (Burgess, 1962). 1960 was also the year in which this author first began planning a body age test. But the most valuable contributors of the early 1960s, in my opinion, were Linder and colleagues from the United States Public Health Service. They were more interested in health than in aging, but their systematic health measures survey of 1962 collected essential data on several thousand adults of all ages, carefully selected as a representative sample of the American people (Linder, 1964, 1966). These confirmed, on a normative American sample, the sensitive age indices of near vision, hearing level at high frequency, systolic blood pressure, and other measures. The early development of my own *Adult Growth Examination* relied heavily on these norms. Subsequent publications by the Public Health analysts pro-

The Adult Growth Examination

vided key data for developing age charts for hearing level (Glorig & Roberts, 1965; Roberts, 1968b), near vision (Roberts, 1964-68), and systolic blood pressure (Gordon, 1964, Roberts, 1975). The vision work was also facilitated by the data collection of Friedenwald (1952) and Bruckner (1959), Rosen *et al.* (1964), and Spoor (1967). The early vision work of Chapanis (1949, 1956) as communicated by many general texts in the early 1960s, was also of great value. By the end of the 1960s my own test was standardized and in practice (Morgan, 1966-72).

In the 1960s, Hollingsworth and colleagues (1965, 1969) did some groundwork on body age testing by defining physiological age with the use of correlations of health measures on Hiroshima subjects. Again the results, published in a journal of biological medicine, were potentially fruitful as Step One in the evolution of a body age test. No Step Two emerged from these authors.

In 1968, Dirken attempted to develop a functional age test based on the abilities of industrial workers. However, he found his approach had difficulty differentiating rapidly aging workers from slowly aging workers.

In 1969, and again in 1972, Comfort assembled an exhaustive 59 measures of aging, ranging from biopsies to gray hairs and including systolic blood pressure (he found the latter to correlate .519 with calendar age). Comfort's battery of tests was much more comprehensive than the one I had developed several years earlier (AGE) but it was this comprehensiveness that limited its application. To be evaluated was time consuming, occasionally painful, and required expensive and sophisticated equipment and personnel. Shortly thereafter, Comfort began his successful publishing career by writing on the "joys of sex," and left England for sunny California. The test battery seems to have fallen into the background.

In 1972, Burr suggested an even more imaginative measure of wellbeing and aging: the monitoring of the electric patterns of life. It was in that year that the call for applied measures of functional age were most frequently expressed. C.L. Rose suggested that we use it to quantify social age; Robert Kastenbaum and colleagues called for a functional age of the self concept; J.L. Fozard described ways in which functional age could be derived from measured abilities and personality; Nuttall called for a functional age based on life expectancy (years from death rather than years from birth). It was Nuttall who was subsequently credited by several gerontology publications as having originated the concept of functional age.

Correlational analysis of age-sensitive factors remains in high gear, ranging from the Nova Scotian Clarke's factorial analysis in 1960 to Furukawa's multiple regression analysis in 1975. The results follow the same pattern: blood pressure, near vision, hearing loss at high frequency, and other measures (see Tables 1 and 2) correlate significantly with calendar age and may be used to predict aging for specific populations by specific formulae.

Despite the periodically published works of Comfort (1969, 1972) and Morgan (1968-1981), the concept of a standardized test for body age continues to be rediscovered. In the late 1970s the late Benjamin Schloss eloquently regaled life extension gatherings with suggestions to develop such a measure, adding creative innovations of his own (such as "Sanar cabinets": Donaldson, 1980). The Linus Pauling Institute collected urine samples from 235 volunteers at a California VA Hospital: computer analysis suggested 30 separate promising age-related constituents (Robinson, 1978). Eventual age scores, based on urine samples, would be used to evaluate the effects of vitamins on aging. More recently, Richard Hochschild, at the UC, Irvine, School of Medicine, is reported to be developing a ten-test battery to determine the effects of deanol and lecithin on aging (Kent, 1980). The Hochschild battery includes reaction time, decision time, shortterm memory, picture recognition, movement speed, vital capacity of the lungs, forced expiratory volume, fingertip vibration acuity, near vision, and high frequency hearing level. The last two, of course, overlap the *Adult Growth Examination.* However, Hochschild omits blood pressure or any other blood measures.

Computerized urine analysis and ten-item test batteries lose the simplicity and speed of the *Adult Growth Examination,* but may yet be the wave of a less populist oriented future. Both approaches have the potential for higher reliability and validity; both should be encouraged. The main advantage of reinventing the wheel is that it may be a better wheel.

At present, however, the only standardized test for general use in the assessment of adult aging is the *Adult Growth Examination.* See the encouraging review of this test by Tom Donaldson of Australian National University, in *Long Life,* 1980.

Test Construction

In developing the *Adult Growth Examination,* a wide variety of

The Adult Growth Examination

physiological measures that correlate with age were evaluated as measures for a brief, painless, reliable and valid test of adult body age. Adaptation to darkness was discarded because of the high cost of reliable measurement equipment and the great length of time-needed to measure it (although it remains an extremely sensitive indicator of aging). Vital capacity was discarded because of equipment cost and weight. Strength and speed tasks were often insufficiently sensitive to pinpoint a body age to the nearest year (as was Lipo-Protein Index). Blood measures and urine measures that involved costly, painful, or time-consuming analysis were discarded. Dental measures lacked sufficient year-specific sensitivity. In the end, the three basic subtests of near vision, hearing loss, and systolic blood pressure were adopted when they were found to be both reliable and valid as well as brief, relatively inexpensive, and comfortable for an examinee to undergo. Extensive and representative norms were available for all of them and, as has been reported, their history is long and respectable.

For those who wish to explore additional promising measures, several are given in the decade charts of Tables 1 and 2. Dark-adaptation techniques, for those with enough time and money, seem to be of superior effectiveness (Domey, 1960; Weale, 1970). Vibration sensitivity continues to have promise (Cosh, 1953) but the most age-sensitive spot is the big toe—and many examinees resent an examiner vibrating this ticklish digit.

Test Standardization

Subtests were standardized by Morgan and colleagues from 1966 to 1972 in Hawaii, New York State and Nova Scotia. Where applicable, the standardized procedures of the Public Health Service examiners (Linder, 1964, 1966) were continued. The present exam procedure has been field tested in a variety of settings for the last seven years with apparent success. By 1998. more than a thousand people had been tested at each decade of life.

Establishment of Norms

Original sources are listed below the decade chart Table 1. Local norms may at times be more appropriate but the nationally representative norms of the tables remain viable for normal usage.

Reliability

To be reliable, a test should give approximately the same results at different times, different places, and under a wide variety of test conditions. The AGE was found to be reliable. In a study of 50 male volunteer Nova Scotians, the test-retest coefficient was .88 with subtest reliability of .93 (NPV), .92 (HL) and .75 (SBP). The results of this study (Morgan & Fevens, 1972) are tabled in Tables 7 and 8, which follow. While the results were highly satisfying, it is still recommended that individual body age scores be re-assessed several times if reliability is essential. The standard error of measurement was found to be about five years; therefore, body age scores less than five years from the calendar age may be due to measurement fluctuation and the person may be considered to be in the normal range for his or her age. For research purposes, significantly rapid or slow agers are considered to be those who vary ± 10 years from their calendar age.

In 1975, Roberts published the results of a new Public Health Service study involving the examination of more than 6,000 persons considered to be representative of the American population. Although the sample tested ranged in age from 18 to 59 and was a more contemporary group than the 1962 sample, the norms were not appropriate to our standardized test. The percentage of the representative probability sample drawn that was actually tested was too low at many age levels to be truly representative. Further, the systolic blood pressure measures were based on only one reading (as opposed to three in 1962) with subsequently poor reliability. Yet, despite all this, Roberts reports the mean values of this 1972 study to differ by a negligible amount from the 1962 study. Systolic blood pressure in 1962 was 121.2 for people 18-44 and 136.5 for people 45-49; in 1972 it was an average 121.3 for those 18-44 and 135.6 for those who were 45-49. The standard error of the mean SBP for the total group was one mm/hg or less, depending on the decade.

It can be concluded that the AGE has solid reliability for testing purposes.

Validity

A valid test of body age would naturally have a strong sensitivity to chronological age. As a predictor of an examinee's calendar age, the full test and all three subtests correlated well: .82 for the full test (subtests in .60s and .72s) (Morgan, 1972). Complete results are pre-

The Adult Growth Examination

sented in Tables 9 & 10 on pages to follow. From Helmholtz & Galton to Clarke (1960), Comfort (1960, 1972) and Furukawa (1975) we have strong correlational confirmation that our three subtests can predict and characterize chronological age.

In longitudinal studies, it has been demonstrated that the scores on subtests continue to decrease at similar rates right through the seventies and, more important, are good predictors of longevity (Palmore, 1974b; Rose *et al.,* 1964-1972). Predictive validity is long documented for some of the subtests (e.g., Helmholtz & presbyopia) when it is longevity that is to be predicted. This is described for our vision test by Bernstein (1945); for systolic blood pressure by Lew (1973) and the 11-year longitudinal study of Granick & Patterson (1971) (nonsmoking and low SBP best survival predictors).

It seems clear that the three measures comprising the overall test of body age have good predictive validity in their individual use. They can be used to predict chronological age or differential survival. With time, the entire test as an entity can also be used for these predictive purposes. In theory, AGE should be a better survival predictor for an individual than insurance company actuarial tables.

People who score 10 or more years over their calendar age can always be told from those scoring 10 years or less; the cosmetic differences are obvious. Further, the examinees know their rapid or slow aging status themselves, although they may understate its magnitude. Comparing such extreme groups is another approach to test validation (Morgan, 1976). Such comparisons are often dramatic examples of the promise of gerontology. I clearly remember examining two Nova Scotian women, both 40 years old; one had a body age of 19 and the other a body age of 60. They both looked their body ages.

Face, content, and predictive validity are respectable for this stage of the test's development. AGE is the most valid (and only) indicator of relative bodily aging in standarized test form available.

Uses

A test of individual body aging may be used for information, enjoyment, self awareness, research and social change. Often, local norms will be needed to maximize its effectiveness. For example, a giant corporation is considering the addition of this test to its health multiphasic battery as used for the workers. Norms for workers in that corporation, at each year of chronological age, would first be gathered and computerized as a data base for individual comparison. Norms would also be needed for cultures much different from ours: Rosen *et al.*, 1964, for example, found hearing loss at 6,000 cps to decline much more gradually with age for Mabaans, a tribe in the Sudan, than has been found to be true for American and European cultures. In our culture, the subtests seem fairly hardy and widely applicable. As a research tool, it has already suggested some important rate of aging differences between ethnic groups or sexes (Morgan, 1968b). Many will use this test to evaluate the effects of special diets, health programs, occupations, and even marriages. One can choose to isolate the many factors leading to premature aging—or exceptional youth. Why do women age most rapidly in their forties? Why do black males average a body-age jump five years higher than white males in their first decade of adult life? These findings must be confirmed and explained before they can be changed. Explorers like MacPherson & Schofield (1971) follow the effect of chronic happiness on aging and determine that lifelong happiness retards the aging process. Wallace *et al.* (1980) used the AGE test to assess the impact of habitual meditation on aging: of 47 meditators averaging 53 chronological years, those meditating for more than five years (24 people) averaged 15 years younger than their birth certificate would predict; the 23 meditators of less than five years' experience showed half that advantage (7 years younger). As with "chronic" happiness, a fairly consistent block of intervention, five years or more, seems to make a substantial difference.

Elkind, using this test as the index, investigated the effects of hypnosis on aging and found that in fact, age yields to hypnosis. Comparisons from test-identified groups of prematurely aged and extremely youthful people are now possible (Morgan, 1977b). Tables 11 and 12 illustrate this. On page 211 is a chart you may wish to use for monitoring your own body age scores over time, or in response to changes in your life style.

The era of self determination is with us, and that self determination includes a decision as to how fast you will allow yourself to age. The *Adult Growth Examination* is an important first step. It lets you know where you stand and it gauges your success when you attempt an improvement.

Recommended general source - books:

Belsky, J. *The Adult Experience.* San Francisco: West/Wadsworth, 1997.
Birren, J.E. (Editor). *Handbook of aging and the individual: psychological and biological aspects.* Chicago: University of Chicago Press, 1959.
Birren, J.E. *The psychology of aging.* Englewood Cliffs, New Jersey: Prentice-Hall, 1964.
Birren, J.E. A brief history of the psychology of aging. I and II. *The Gerontologist,* 1961.
Birren, J.E. Psychological aspects of aging. *Annual Review of Psychology,* 1960.
Birren, J.E., Imus, H.A., and Windle, W.F. (Editors). *The process of aging and the nervous system.* Oxford: Blackwell Scientific Publications, 1959.
Birren, J.E. and Schaie, K.W. (Editors). *Handbook of the Psychology of Aging.* New York: Van Nostrand Reinhold, 1977.
Birren, J.E. and Wall, P.D. Age changes in conduction velocity, refractory period, number of fibers, connective tissue space and blood vessels in sciatic nerve of rats. *Journal of Comparative Neurology,* 1956.
Birren, J.E.; Kenyon, G.M.; Ruth, J. editors. *Aging & Biography: Explorations in Adult Development.* New York: Springer Pub. Co., 1996.
Cohen, Stanley. Sleep Thieves. New York: Free Press, 1997.
Dean, Ward. Biological Aging Measurement, 2nd edition. Los Angeles, CA, Center for Bio Gerontology, 1988.
Duran, Eduardo; Duran, Bonnie. Native American Postcolonial Psychology. Albany, New York, State University of New York Press, 1995.
Gruman, G.J. *History of Ideas about the Prolongation of Life.* Stamford, N.H., Ayer co. Pub., 1977. (Out of print, but available from instructor.)
Fried, S.B. & Mehrotra, C.M. *Aging & Diversity.* Washington D.C., Taylor & Francis, 1997, Pb.
Heynen, J. One Hundren Over 100. Golden, CO., Fulcrum Pub., 1990.

Kent, S. *The Life Extension Revolution.* New York: Morrow, 1980.

LeFrancois, Guy. The Life Span, 6th edition. San Francisco: Wadsworth, 1999.

Luce, G.G. Longer Life More Joy: Techniques for Enhancing Health, Happiness and Inner Vision. North Hollywood, CA, Newcastle Publishing Co., 1992.

McAdams, D.P.; DeSt. Aubin, E. editors. Generativity & Adult Development. Washington, D.C., APA, 1998.

Newman, S.; Ward, C.R.; Smith, T.B.; Wilson, J. Intergenerational Programs: Past, Present and Future. Washington, D.C., Taylor & Francis, 1997, Pb.

Nordus, I.H.; Vandenbos, G.R.; Berg, S.; Fromholt, P. editors. Clinical Geropsychology. Washington, D.C., APA, 1998.

Poon, L.W. *Aging in the 198 Os: Psychological Issues.* Washington, D.C.: American Psychological Association, 1980.[1]

Robbins, T. Jitterbug Perfume. New York: Bantam Books, 1990, Pb.

Scogin, F.; Prohaska, M. Aiding Older Adults with Memory Complaints. Sarasota, Flordia, Professional Resource Exchange, 1993, Pb.

Sheehy, Gail. New Passages. New York, Ballantine Books (Trd Pap), 1996.

Stoller, E.P.; Gibson, R.C. *Worlds of Difference: Inequity in the Aging Experience, 2nd edition.* Thousand Oaks, CA, Pine Forge Press, 1997.

Storandt, M.; Vandenbos, G.R. editor. *The Adult Years: Continuity and Change.* Washington, D.C., APA 1989.

---

[1]*Note: Poon's book Aging in the 1980s is an excellent summary of research on aging from the psychological point of view with one significant omission: no chapters focus on the systematic measurement of human aging as a general process. The mystery of this blind spot may be explained by Welford's last summarizing chapter, which states: "Functional age of individuals can, therefore, be assessed only for particular tasks: One individual may be functionally older than another for one task but functionally younger for a different task. No meaningful overall index of functional age is possible" (p. 618). The strong significant correlations between measures, and the subsequent mortality for each measure, used in body age measurement batteries suggests a much more optimistic picture than Welford portrays ... perhaps Aging in the 21st Century will be more up to date.*

The Adult Growth Examination

Whitbourne, S.K. *The Aging Individual: Physical & Psychological Perspectives.* New York., Springer Publishing Co., 1996.

Wolman, B.B. *Handbook of General Psychology.* Englewood Cliffs, New Jersey: Prentice-Hall, 1973. Developmental Psychology Ch. 42 on aging.

Zarit, S.; Knight, B.G., editors. *A Guide to Psychotherpy & Aging: Effective Clinical Interventions in a Life State Context.* Washington, D.C., APA, 1998

Suggested readings by R.F. Morgan on applied gerontology and the measurement of human aging:

"An Introduction to Applied Gerontology." *Long Term Care and Health Services Administration Quarterly,* 1977, *1,* 168-178.

"The Adult Growth Examination: Follow-up Note on Comparisons between Rapidly Aging Adults and Slowly Aging Adults as De fined by Body Age." *InterAmerican Journal of Psychology,* 1977, *11,* 10-13.

Conquest of Aging: Modern Measurement and Intervention. Second edition, Pueblo, Colorado: Applied Gerontology Communications, 1977. This edition is now sold out but copies are available in many university libraries or from the author.

Measurement of Human Aging in Applied Gerontology. Dubuque, Iowa: Kendall/Hunt; Toronto: Holt, 1981.

Interventions in Applied Gerontology. Dubuque, Iowa: Kendall/Hunt; Toronto: Holt, 1981.

Decades of Research and Practice with the Adult Growth Examination" in HUMAN BIOLOGIC AGE DETERMINATION (A.K. Balin, editor), Ann Arbor: CRC Press, 1994.

Training the Time Sense. Fair Oaks, CA: Morgan Foundation Publishers 1999

Growing Younger

REPRINTED TABLES

Table 7. *Adult Growth Examination (AGE)* Test-Retest Correlations For 50 Males With Chronological Ages of 20 to 70 Years

AGE Varibles	Raw Score r	Age Score r
Subtest 1: Hearing Loss	.95*	.92*
Subtest 2: Near Vision	.93*	.93*
Subtest 3: Systolic blood pressure	.79*	.75*
Median of subtests 1 & 2	- - -	.95*
Median of subtests 1 & 3	- - -	.81*
Median of subtests 2 & 3	- - -	.83*
AGE total score: Median of all subtests	- - -	.88*

*p < .01

From Morgan & Fevens, 1994

Table 8. Selected *Adult Growth Examination (AGE)* Correlations Comparisons

AGE Variables	Raw Score r*	Age Score r*
A. Correlation with chronological age:		
Subtest 1: Hearing Loss	.68 (.66)	.76 (.69)
Subtest 2: Near Vision	.73 (.57)	.84 (.78)
Subtest 3: Systolic blood pressure	.55 (.69)	.81 (.82)
AGE total score (Median 1, 2, 3)	- - -	.81 (.82)
B. Subtest inter-correlations:		
Subtest 1: Hearing Loss	.66 (.46)	.73 (.63)
Subtest 2: Near Vision	.38 (.47)	.43 (.52)
Subtest 3: Systolic blood pressure	.59 (.43)	.60 (.53)
C. Correlation of subtests with AGE total score:		
Subtest 1: Hearing Loss	.67 (.65)	.73 (.74)
Subtest 2: Near Vision	.84 (.64)	.89 (.81)
Subtest 3: Systolic blood pressure	.81 (.84)	.82 (.85)

Note: All correlation in parentheses are based on a validation sample of 107 Nova Scotia male and female volunteers aged 20 to 70 years. They are presented above for comparison with correlations based exclusively on the 50 Nova Scotia male volunteers aged 20 to 70 years who were tested and retested for the present reliability study. The former sample's date derive from Morgan 1970b.
*p < .01 for every product-moment correlation in the table

From Morgan & Fevens, 1994

Table 9. Selected Analyses of *Adult Growth Examination (AGE)* Scores of Nova Scotians of Both Sexes Aged 20 to 70 Years

Selected Analyses	Raw Scores	Age Scores	n
Correlation with chronological age:			
AGE total score for both sexes	------	r is .82**	107
AGE total score for females only	------	r is .83**	56
AGE total score for males only	------	r is .81**	51
Subtest 1: Hearing Loss	r is .66**	r is .69**	107
Subtest 2: Near Vision	r is .57**	r is .78**	101
Subtest 3: Systolic blood pressure	r is .69**	r is .67**	105
Median of subtests 1 & 2	------	r is .69**	101
Median of subtests 1 & 3	------	r is .78**	106
Median of subtests 2 & 3	------	r is .66**	101
Subtest Intercorrelations:			
Subtest 1 & 2	r is .46**	r is .63**	101
Subtest 1 & 3	r is .47**	r is .52**	106
Subtest 2 & 3	r is .43**	r is .53**	101
Correlation with AGE total score:			
Subtest 1: Hearing Loss	r is .65**	r is .74** M/I	107
Subtest 2: Near Vision	r is .64**	r is .81** M/I	101
Subtest 3: Systolic blood pressure	r is .84**	r is .85** M/I	106
Median of subtests 1 & 2	------	r is .85**	101
Median of subtests 1 & 3	------	r is .89**	106
Median of subtests 2 & 3	------	r is .93**	101

**p < .01 for every product-moment correlation in the table

From Morgan, 1994

Table 10. Further Analyses of *Adult Growth Examination (AGE)* Scores of Nova Scotians of Both Sexes Aged 20 to 70 Years

Analysis	Results	
Standard error is estimate (in years) of chronological age:		
AGE total score for both sexes	S.E.E. is 9.30 years,	n = 107
Subtest 1: Hearing Loss	S.E.E. is 11.23 years,	n = 107
Subtest 2: Near Vision	S.E.E. is 8.11 years,	n = 101
Subtest 3: Systolic blood pressure	S.E.E. is 14.33 years,	n = 106
Median of subtests 1 & 2	S.E.E. is 7.61 years,	n = 101
Median of subtests 1 & 3	S.E.E. is 10.05 years,	n = 106
Median of subtests 2 & 3	S.E.E. is 8.87 years,	n = 101
Medians per item (M/I) frequencies (Morgan, 1964) by subtest:		
Subtest 1: Hearing Loss	M/I is 21*	n = 101
Subtest 2: Near Vision	M/I is 44*	n = 101
Subtest 3: Systolic blood pressure	M/I is 36*	n = 101

Distribution of AGE scores in relation to chronological age:
BA[1] = CA 7% sample BA older than CA: 50% sample BA younger than CA: 43% BA within ± 5 years of CA: 47% of samples: BA within ± 10 years CA: 67% sample.
Average difference in years between BA and CA: 8 years.

Individual estimates of body age (EBA):
For full sample (N=107) median EBA is 35 years: median BA & median CA: 40 years.
Average difference in years between EBA and BA is 7½ years, Correct EBAs: 7%.

Sex differences: none of the above analyses demonstrated significant sex differences.

---

[1] –BA is Body Age (total AGE score)   *$p < .05$ (Morgan, 1964)

From Morgan, 1994

Table 11. Analyses of Slow, Normal, and Rapid Age Rate Groups of Nova Scotians of Both Sexes: Age in Years by Birth (CA), by Measurement (BA), be Self Estimate (EA)

Age rate group:	"Young" Slow Agers	Normal Agers	"Older" Rapid Agers
Number of people	9	18	10
Average CA:	53	52	46
Average BA:	38	52	61
Average EA:	47	52	47
CA range:	40-60	40-60	40-60
BA range:	19-49	35-65	53-71+
EA range:	30-60	32-60	35-55
Mean difference from CA:			
BA-CA:	-15	0	+15
EA-CA:	-6	0	+1
Mean difference from BA:			
CA-BA:	+15	0	-15
EA-BA:	+9	0	+14

Additional note on EA: using CA as a reference point, 0% of the "young" slow agers estimated themselves *older* than their birth age (normal agers estimated themselves older 17% group) while "older" rapid agers estimated themselves *younger* than their birth age in only 20% of their group (normal agers estimated themselves younger 44% group). Thus incidence of mistaken direction of aging was low in both slow and rapid age rate groups.

From Morgan, 1994

Table 12. Analyses of Slow, Normal, and Rapid Age Rate Groups of Nova Scotians of Both Sexes: Selected Differentiating Factors From Questionnaire Data

Age rate group:	"Young" Slow Agers	Normal Agers	"Older" Rapid Agers
Number of people	9	18	10
% Females	44	56	80
Median Annual Income:	$6,000.00	$6,000.00	$3,881.00*
Maximum Annual Income:	$20,000.00	$15,000.00	$6,000.00
Lifetime Happiness:	78%	67%	40%
Present Happiness:	44%	44%	50%
First born:	22%	22%	56%
Median number of Cigarette packs smoked Per week over lifetime:	0	0	2

Undifferentiating factors: marital status, marital satisfaction, number of children, number of occupants in house, religion, church attendance, present health, lifetime health, physical appearance, personal adjustment, punctuality, job satisfaction, present happiness, alcohol consumption, intercourse frequency.

*$p < .05$; Efficiency percentage (Morgan, 1968a) for differentiating rapid agers from normal group is 90% and from slow agers is also 90%.

From Morgan, 1994

BIBLIOGRAPHY

American Heart Association. Major risk factors in heart disease. *World Almanac & Book of Facts 1976.* New York; Newspaper Enterprise Association, 1975.

Belsky, J. *The Adult Experience.* San Francisco: West/Wadsworth, 1997.

Benjamin, H. Outline of a method to estimate the biological age with special reference to the role of sexual functions. *International Journal of Sexology,* 1949, *3,* 34-37.

Bernstein, F. Law of physiologic aging as derived from long range data in refraction of the human eye. *Archives of Ophthalmology,* 1945, *45,* 378-388.

Birren, J.E. (Editor). *Handbook of aging and the individual: psychological and biological aspects.* Chicago: University of Chicago Press, 1959.

Birren, J.E.; Kenyon, G.M.; Ruth, J. editors. *Aging & Biography: Explorations in Adult Development.* New York: Springer Pub. Co., 1996.

Bruckner, R. Uber methoden longitudinaler alternsforschung am auge. *Ophthalmologica,* 1959, *138, 59—75.*

Burgess, E.W. A comparison of the interdisciplinary findings of the study of objective criteria of aging. In C. Tibbits & W. Donahue (Editors) *Social and psychological aspects of aging—aging around the world: Proceedings of the Fifth Congress of the International Association of Gerontology in San Francisco, 1960.* New York: Columbia University Press, 1962.

Burr, H.S. Blueprint for immortality: the electric patterns of life. London: Neville Spearman, Ltd., 1972.

Chapanis, A., Garver, W., & Morgan, C.T. *Applied experimental psychology* New York: Wiley, 1949. (Cf. Chapanis chapter on vision in C.T. Morgan, Editor, *Introduction to psychology,* New York: McGraw-Hill, 1956, pp. 449-479.)

Clarke, I. The aging dimension: a factorial analysis of individual differences with age on psychological and physiological measurements. Journal of Gerontology, 1960, 15, 183—187.

Cohen, Stanley. Sleep Thieves. New York: Free Press, 1997.

Comfort, A. Measuring the human aging rate. Mechanisms of Aging & Development, 1972, 1, 101—110.

Comfort, A. Test battery to measure aging rate in men. Lancet, 1969, 2, 1411.

Corday, E. & Vyden, K. Electronic monitors in medicine. Journal of the American Association of Medical Instrumentation, 1966, 7.

Corso, J.F. Age and sex differences in pure-tone thresholds. Journal of the Acoustical Society of America, 1959, 3 1, 498—507.

Cosh, J.A. Studies on the nature of the vibrations sense. Clinical Science, 1953, 12, 131—273.

Dean, Ward. Biological Aging Measurement, 2nd edition. Los Angeles, CA, Center for Bio Gerontology, 1988.

Dirken, J.M. The functional age of industrial workers. Mens en ondernem, 1968a, 22, 226-273.

Dirken, J.M. A tentative judgment about the "yardstick" for functional age. Mens en ondernem, 1968b, 22, 342—351.

Domey, R., McFarland, R. & Chadwock, E. Threshold and rate of dark adaptation as a function of age and time. Human Factors, 1960, 2, 109-119.

Donaldson, T.K. Books: Manual for the Adult Growth Examination Long Life, 1980, 4(2), #17, 43.

Duran, Eduardo; Duran, Bonnie. Native American Postcolonial Psychology. Albany, New York, State University of New York Press, 1995.

Elkind, L. Effects of hypnosis on the process of aging. Unpublished doctoral dissertation, California School of Professional Psychology, San Francisco, 1972.

Florey, C. & Acheson, R.M. Blood pressure as it relates to physique, blood glucose, and serum cholesterol. Washington, D.C.: Public Health Service Pub. 1000, series 11, no. 34, 1969.

Fozard, J.L. Predicting age in the adult years from psychological assessments of abilities and personality. Aging and Human Development, 1972, 3, 175—182.

Bibliography

Fried, S.B. & Mehrotra, C.M. *Aging & Diversity*. Washington D.C., Taylor & Francis, 1997, Pb.

Friedenwald, J.S. The eye. In A.I. Lansing (Editor) *Cowdry's problems of aging, 3rd edition*. Baltimore: Williams & Wilkins, 1952.

Furukawa, T., Inoue, M., Kajiya, F., Inada, H., Takasugi, S., Fukui, S., Takeda, H., & Abe, H. Assessment of biological age by multiple regression analysis. *Journal of Gerontology*, 1975, 30, 422—434.

Galton, F. *Inquiries into human faculty and its development, 2nd edition*. New York: Dutton, 1907.

Garst, C.C. *Blood glucose levels in adults*. Washington, D.C.: Public Health Service publication 1000, series 11, no. 18, 1966.

Gavurin, E.I. & Pockell, N.E. Comparison of bare handed and glove handed finger dexterity. *Perceptual & Motor Skills*, 1963, 16, 246.

Glorig, A. & Roberts, I. *Hearing levels of adults by age and sex*. Washington, D.C.: Public Health Service publication 1000, series 11, no. U, 1965.

Gordon, T. *Blood pressure of adults by age and sex*. Washington, D.C.: Public Health Service publication 1000, series 11, no. 4, 1964a.

Gordon, T. *Blood pressure of adults by race and area*. Washington, D.C.: Public Health Service publication 1000, series 11, no. 5, 1964b.

Gordon, T. & Devine, B. *Hypertension and hypertensive heart disease in adults*. Washington, D.C.: Public Health Service publication 1000, series 11, no. 13, 1966.

Granick, S. & Patterson, R.D. *Human aging II: an eleven year follow-up biomedical and behavioural study*. Rockville, Maryland: USDHEW National Institute of Mental Health publication (HSM) 71-9037, 1971.

Gruman, G.J. *History of Ideas about the Prolongation of Life*. Stamford, N.H., Ayer co. Pub., 1977. (Out of print, but available from instructor.)

Heidemann, R. *Presbyopie und Lebensdauer*. Goettingen: Inaugural Dissertation, 1932.

Heynen, J. One Hundren Over 100. Golden, CO., Fulcrum Pub., 1990.

Hollingsworth, D.R., Hollingsworth, J.W., Bogitch, S. Neuromuscular tests of aging in Hiroshima survivors. Journal of Gerontology, 1969, 24, 276—283.

Hollingsworth, J.W., Hashizume, A., & Jablon, S. Correlations between tests of aging in Hiroshima subjects—an attempt to de fine physiological age. Yale Journal of Biological Medicine, 1965, 38, 11.

Jalavisto, E. The role of simple tests measuring speed and performance in the assessment of biological vigour: a factorial study of elderly women. In A. Welford & J. Birren (Editors) Behavior, aging, and the nervous system. Springfield, Illinois: Thomas, 1965. Pp. 13—25.

Jalavisto, E. & Makkonen, T. On the assessment of biological age: I. Factor analysis of physiological measurements in old and young women. Annals of the Academy of Fenn. Science, 1963a. 100, 1—38.

Jalavisto, E. & Makkonen, T. On the assessment of biological age: II. A factoral study of aging in postmenopausal women. Annals of the Academy of Fenn. Science, 1963b, 101, 1—15.

Johnson, E.S., Kelly, I.E., & Van Kirk, L.E. Selected dental findingsforadults. Washington, D.C.: Public Health Service publication 1000, series 11, no. 7, 1965.

Jones, H.B., Gofman, J.W., Lindgren, F.T., Lyon, T.P., & Strisower, B. Lipoproteins in atherosclerosis. American Journal of Medicine, 1951, 11, 358—380.

Kastenbaum, R., Derbin, V., Sabatini, P., & Artt, S. "The ages of me:" toward personal and interpersonal definitions of functional aging. Aging and Human Development, 1972, 3, 197—212.

Kelly, J.E., Van Kirk, L.E., & Garst, C.C. Decayed, missing, and filled teeth in adults. Washington, D.C.: Public Health Service publication 1000, series 11, no. 23, 1969.

Kelly, J.E. & Van Kirk, L.E. Peridontal disease in adults. Washington, D.C.: Public Health Service publication 1000, series 11, no. 12, 1965. Kent, S. The life extension revolution. New York: Morrow, 1980.

LeFrancois, Guy. The Life Span, 6th edition. San Francisco: Wadsworth, 1999.
Lew, E.A. High blood pressure, other risk factors, and longevity: the insurance viewpoint. American Journal of Medicine, 1973, 55, 281—294.
Linder, F.E. The health of the American people. ScientificAmerican, 1966, 2 14(6), 21-29.
Linder, F.E. Cycle I of the health examination survey: sample and response. Washington, D.C.: Public Health Service publication 1000, series 11, no. 1, 1964.
Luce, G.G. Longer Life More Joy: Techniques for Enhancing Health, Happiness and Inner Vision. North Hollywood, CA, Newcastle Publishing Co., 1992.
MacPherson, K. & Schofield, M. Happiness is a warm bed. Unpublished research at Acadia University, Wolfville, Nova Scotia, 1971.
McAdams, D.P.; DeSt. Aubin, E. editors. Generativity & Adult Development. Washington, D.C., APA, 1998.
Moore, F.E. & Gordon, T. Serum cholesterol levels in adults. Washington, D.C.: Public Health Service publication 1000, series 11, no. 22, 1967.
Morgan, R.F. Conquest of aging: modern measurement & intervention. Second edition. Pueblo, Colorado: Applied Gerontology Communications 1977a. Two more recent (1981) releases listed at end of bibliography.
Morgan, R.F. The Adult Growth Examination: follow-up note on comparisons between rapidly aging adults and slowly aging adults as defined by body age. Inter-American Journal of Psychology, 1977, 11, 10—13.
Morgan, R.F. An introduction to applied gerontology. Long Term Care & Health Services Administration Quarterly, 1977c, 1, 168—178.
Morgan, R.F. The ADULT GROWTH EXAMINATION (AGE): Manual for a compact standarized test of individual aging. Second edition (revised). Pueblo, Colorado: Psychology Department, University of Southern Colorado, 1976.
Morgan, R.F. The *Adult Growth Examination:* validation, analysis, and cross-cultural utility of a brief compact test of individual

aging. *InterAmerican Journal of Psychology (Revista Interamericana de Psicologia)*, 1972, *6*, 245—254.

Morgan, R.F. *The Adult Growth Examination (AGE):* Manual for a compact standardized test of individual aging. Un published manual: 1st edition. San Francisco: California School of Professional Psychology, October, 1971.

Morgan, R.F. How old are you, really: techniques for assessing differential aging. *The Canadian Magazine,* 1970, February 28, 2—4.

Morgan, R.F. Are you older than you think? *Science Digest,* 1969b, *66*, August, 20—21.

Morgan, R.F. *The Adult Growth Examination: standardization and - normative data for male and female adults in New York and Nova Scotia.* Unpublished study at Acadia University, Wolfville, Nova Scotia, 1969c.

Morgan, R.F. The need for greater use of efficiency percentages to supplement reports of statistical significance. *Perceptual & Motor Skills,* 1968a, *27,* 338.

Morgan, R.F. Memory and the senile psychoses: a follow-up note. *Psychological Reports,* 1967, *20,* 733—734.

Morgan, R.F. The *Hawaii Age Test (HAT)* for bodily aging in adults: standardization and reliability of measures. Alias: the effects of rate and duration of consumption of alcoholic beverages on bodily aging. Unpublished research proposal at Hawaii State Hospital, Kaneohe, 1966.

Morgan, R.F. Note on the psychopathology of senility: senescent defense against the threat of death. *Psychological Reports,* 1965, *16,* 305-306.

Morgan, R.F. the MII frequencies: a quick and computation free nonparametric method of test item evaluation. *Psychological Reports,* 1965, *14,* 723—728.

Morgan, R.F. & Fevens, S.K. Reliability of the *Adult Growth E x - amination:* a standardized test of individual aging. *Perceptual & Motor Skills,* 1972, 34, 415—419.

Murray, I.M. Assessment of physiological age by combination of several criteria: vision, hearing, blood pressure, and muscle force. Journal of Gerontology, 1951, 6, 120—126.

Newman, S.; Ward, C.R.; Smith, T.B.; Wilson, J. Intergenerational Programs: Past, Present and Future. Washington, D.C., Taylor & Francis, 1997, Pb.

Bibliography

Nordus, I.H.; Vandenbos, G.R.; Berg, S.; Fromholt, P. editors. Clinical Geropsychology. Washington, D.C., APA, 1998.
Nuttall, R.L. The strategy of functional age research. Aging & Human Development, 1972, 3, 149—152.
Palmore, E. Predicting longevity: a new method. In E. Palmore (Editor) Normal aging II: reports from the Duke Longitudinal Studies 1970— 1973. Durham, North Carolina: Duke Univesity Press, 1974a.
Palmore, E. (Editor). Normal aging II: report from the Duke Longitudinal Studies 1970-1973. Durham, N. Carolina: Duke University Press, 1974b.
Palmore, E. (Editor). Normal aging: reports from the Duke Longitudinal Study 1955—1969. Durham, N. Carolina: Duke University Press, 1970.
Palmore, E. Physical, mental, and social factors in predicting longevity. The Gerontologist, 1969a, 9, 103—108.
Palmore, E. Predicting longevity: a follow-up controlling for age. The Gerontologist, 1969b, 9, 247—250.
Poon, L.W. Aging in the 1980s: psychological issues. Washington, D.C.: American Psychological Association, 1980.
Robbins, T. Jitterbug Perfume. New York: Bantam Books, 1990, Pb.
Roberts, J. Blood pressure of persons 18-74 years in the United States 1971—1972. Rockville, Maryland: Public Health Service publication HRA 75-1632, 1975.
Roberts, J. Hearing status and ear examination findings among adults: Washington, D.C.: Public Health Service Publication 1000, series 11, no. 32, 1968 a.
Roberts, J. Monocular-binocular visual acuity of adults. Washinton, D.C.: Public Health Service publication 1000, series 11, no. 30, 1968b.
Roberts, J. Binocular visual acuity of adults by region and selected demographic characteristics. Washington, D.C.: Public Health Service publication 1000, series 11, no. 25, 1967.
Roberts, J. Weight by height and age of adults. Washington, D.C.: Public Health Service publication 1000, series 11, no. 14, 1966.
Roberts, J. Binocular visual acuity of adults. Washington, D.C.: Public Health Service publication 1000, series 11, no. 3, 1964.
Roberts, J. & Bayliss, D. Hearing levels of adults by race, region, and area of residence. Washington, D.C.: Public Health Service

publication 1000, series 11, no. 31, 1968a.

Roberts, J. & Cohrssen, 1. Hearing levels of adults by education, income, and occupation. Washington, D.C.: Public Health Service publication 1000, series 11, no. 31, 1968a.

Roberts, J. & Cohrssen, J. History and examination findings related to visual acuity among adults. Washington, D.C.: Public Health Service publication 1000, series 11, no. 28, 1968b.

Robinson, A.B. Why do we age? Can we diminish the rate and debilitating effect of aging? Linus Pauling Institute Newsletter, 1978, 1, (June), 3.

Rose, C.L. Measurement of social age. Aging & Human Development, 1972, 3, 153.

Rose, C.L. Social factors in longevity. The Gerontologist, 1964, 4, 27—37.

Rose, C.L. & Bell, B. Predicting longevity: methodology and critique. Lexington, Mass.: Heath, 1971.

Rose, C.L., Enslein, K., & Nuttall, R.L. Univariate & multivariate findings from a longevity study. Proceedings of the 20th annual meeting of the Gerontological Society, 196, 42.

Rosee, B.C. Untersuchungen uber das normale Harvermogen in der verscheidenen Lebensaltern unter besonderer Berucksichtigung der Prufung mit dem Autiometer. Zeitschrift fuer Laryngoligie, Rhinologie, Otologie und ihre Grenzgebiete, 1953, 32, 414—420.

Rosen, S., Plester, D., El-Mofty, E., & Rosen, H.V. High frequency audiometry in presbycusis: a comparative study of the Mabaan tribe in the Sudan with urban populations. Archives of Otolaryngology, 1964, 79, 18—32.

Scogin, F.; Prohaska, M. Aiding Older Adults with Memory Complaints. Sarasota, Flordia, Professional Resource Exchange, 1993, Pb.

Sheehy, Gail. New Passages. New York, Ballantine Books (Trd Pap), 1996.

Spoor, A. Presbycusis values in relations to noise induced hearing loss. *International audiology,* 1967, *6,* 48—57.

Steinhaus, H. Untersuchungen ueber den Zusammenhang von Presbyopie und Lebensdauer, unter Beruecksichtigung der Todesursachen. *Archiven fuer Augenkunde,* 1932, *105,* 731—760.

Stoller, E.P.; Gibson, R.C. *Worlds of Difference: Inequity in the Ag-*

Bibliography

ing Experience, 2nd edition. Thousand Oaks, CA, Pine Forge Press, 1997.

Storandt, M.; Vandenbos, G.R. editor. *The Adult Years: Continuity and Change.* Washington, D.C., APA 1989.

Walk, D. E. Finger dexterity of the pressure suited subject on the Purdue Pegboard Dexterity Test. *United States Air Force AMRC-TDR no. 64—41,* 1965.

Wallace, R.K., Jacobs, D.E., & Harrington, B. Reversal of biological aging in subjects practicing the transcendental meditation technique. Paper delivered to the 36th annual meeting of the American Geriatrics Society, April, 1979.

Weale, R.A. The eye and measurement of aging rate. *Lancet,* 1970, *1,* 147. Wolman, B.B. (Editor). *Handbook of general psychology.* Englewood Cliffs, New Jersey: Prentice-Hall, 1973. Ch. 42 Developmental Psy- chology by Buhler, Keith-Spiegel, & Thomas.

Whitbourne, S.K. *The Aging Individual: Physical & Psychological Perspectives.* New York., Springer Publishing Co., 1996.

Zarit, S.; Knight, B.G., editors. *A Guide to Psychotherpy & Aging: Effective Clinical Interventions in a Life State Context.* Washington, D.C., APA, 1998

More recent releases:

*Morgan, R.F. *Measurement of Human Aging in Applied Gerontology.* Dubuque, Iowa: Kendall Hunt, 1981; Toronto: Holt, 1981. Paperback.

*Morgan, R.F. *Interventions in Applied Gerontology.* Dubuque, Iowa: Kendall Hunt, 1981; Toronto: Holt, 1981. Paperback.

Growing Younger

INDEX

Abkhasians, 81-105
  arteriosclerosis, 83, 90
  comparison with West, 94, 103-105
  diet, 90-92
  folk medicine, 94
  genetic selectivity, 81
  Kinship structure, 90, 91
  marriage, 85
  roles of women, 85, 96
  sexual energy, 85
  temporal integration, 93-95
  work habits, 87-89
Adult Growth Examination (AGE), 9-27, 31-40, 108, 219-254
  anecdotes, 19-21
  auxiliary measures, 19
  background, 239-243
  basic measures, 17, 19
  blacks, in relation to whites, 13, 251
  body age tables, 228-237
  chronological age, 16, 17, 24, 238
  economic bracket, 23
  equipment, 15, 220, 221
  general suggestions, 239, 240
  happiness, 23, 107 245
  high-frequency hearing, 15
  how. to administer, 14-18
  hypnosis, 24, 25-37, 246
  interpreting, 224
  monitor record, 227
  national health survey, 13
  near-point vision, 15
  Nova Scotia study, 21-23
  presbyopia, 10, 11, 252
  reliability, 244
  score sheet, 230
  scoring, 228
  sex differences, 13
  smoking, 23
  systolic blood pressure, 15
  test construction, 242
  test procedure, 221-224
  test standardization; 243
  time requirements, 224
  uses, 245
  validity, 244
Advertising, 2, 28, 29
Aging, xiii-xvi
  definition of, xii
  process of, xiii-xvi
Alcohol, 55, 60, 61, 66, 142, 146
Altitude, 79, 80, 109, 110
Anniversary Neurosis, 47, 48
Anti-Oxidents, 64, 65, 67, 166
Anti-Pyretics, 71
Applied Gerontology, xi, xiii
Attitude, 106-110
Autonomic Nervous System, 29

Baller; W., viii, 127
Bayley, N., 167
Bender, L., 165
Benet, S., vii, 79-106, 123
Benjamin, H., 249
Bergman, A., 152
Bernstein, F., 11, 242, 245
Biofeedback, 47, 112, 116, 117, 121
Birren, J., viii, 239
Birth, 109, 120, 121, 158, 159
Body Temperature, 70-73, 117
Body Weight, 5, 6, 61
Brain Weight, 156

Caffeine, 55, 61, 66, 142, 146
Cancer, 51, 62, 70, 147
Cantor, Dr., 53
Casler, L., vii, 40-44
Cheek, D., vii, 45-47, 170
Child Development Norms, 166, 167
Clark, L., 159
Comfort, A., viii, 240, 241, 244
Cooper, L., viii, 131, 132
Cummings, N., ix, 50

265

DNA, 60
Dawson, A., viii, 127
Death, xi, 2, 123
   expectation of, 43, 48, 49
deVries, H.A., 118, 119
Deyl, Z., 58
Diets, 54, 58, 65, 67, 155
Doll, E., 169

ESP, 51
Einstein, A., 131, 254
Elkind, L., vii, 25-38, 149, 150, 151, 170, 247
Erickson, M., viii, 132, 148
Esdaile, J., 31
Exercise, 118, 123

Frank, B., 62
Freud, S., 128, 148

Galton, F., vii, 9, 248, 249, 255
Genetics, 170
Gerontologists' Diets, 63
Ginseng, 61
Graphotherapy, 30
Guided Imagery, 170

Harman D., viii, 62
Harwood, E., 129
Hayflick, L., 165
Heart Rate, 73, 117
Helmholtz, H., viii, 9, 239, 245
Hochschild, R., 241, 242
Holden, M., 74
Hunzas, 105
Hypnosis, 26-40, 48-50, 52, 247
   Adult Growth Examination, 34-40, 219, 247
   aging, 40
   birth, 48, 49, 114
      body temperature, 72
      cancer, 51
      definition of, 28
      induction, 33, 35
      memory, 48, 49
      stress reduction, 48

      suggestion, relation to, 48
      surgery, 33
      temporal experience, 134-143
      unconcscious mind, 37
      utilization, 33

Iatrogenic Hazards, 153-171
   birth, 158, 159
   defeatism, 161, 163
   disorders, 153, 154
   families, 157, 158
   radiation, 159-160
   school, 158

Jarvik, L., viii, 169
Jones, H.B., 244
Juricova-Horakova, M., 58

Kunz, P., 48
   Leaf, A., viii, 123
LeBoyer, F., viii, 107, 120, 158
LeCron, L., 48
Linder, F.E., 10, 239, 243
Lipo-Protein Index, 239
Longevity, 3, 4
   predictors of, 7
   program for, 173
Love, 127, 128
Luce, G., 107, 118

Marriage, 127, 128
McCay, C., viii, 55, 59, 70
   McCay Method, The, 55-59, 64, 70
Meditation, 117, 121, 247
Mencken, H.L., 124
Miller, N., 29
Murry, I.M., viii, 239

Neill, A.S., 113
Nicotine, 59, 65, 155

Index

Nuttall, R.L., 246

Odens, M., 61
Orr, L., 159
Osteoporosis, 63

Palmore, E., viii, 244
Passwater, D., 5, 59, 64-66
Pauling, L., 61
Phoenix Lodge, 171, 172
Pierce, R.V., 53, 54, 62
Primal Therapy, 74
Pritikin, N., viii, 64, 73
Psychosomatic Medicine, 107
Purpose, 127-130

RNA, 60
Rank, 0., 158
Rapoport, D., 120
  Retirement, 124, 125, 130
  Rose, C.L., x, 241, 245
  Rosenberg, B., x, 69
  Rush, B., 127

SAGE, 108, 118, 125
Salt, 64, 155
Schmeidler, G., 49
Schoenfeld, G., 40
  Scientific Method, xvi
  Self-Fulfilling Prophecy, 28, 39, 40, 43, 44, 46, 48, 117, 156, 168, 173
  Self-Programming, 42-51
  Selye H., viii, 108
  Senility, xi, 121, 149
  Sex, 123-127, 130
  Sheilds, E., 119
  Shock N., 169
  Shunamitism, 126
  Sichinava, G.N., 83, 86, 87
  Sleep, 75-77
  Socrates, 30
  Steinhaus, H., 10, 11, 243

Strehler, B., viii, 69
Sugar, 156;
  see also Diets

Temperature, Body, 70-777, 117
Temporal Conditioning, 154, 155
Third Force Psychology, 111
Time Condensation, 132
Time Expansion, 132
Tolstoy, L., 100
Transpersonal Psychology, 112-122
  educational co-operatives, 114-118
  parapsychology, 120
  purpose, 113
  techniques, 116
  view on mental institutions, 114

U.S. Public Health Service, 5, 10, 243

Vitamins, 59-61, 65-69, 78, 163, 168
Vonnegut, K., 131

Warner, S.J., 44
Williams, R., 59, 60
Work, 121, 122, 126

Yoga, 117, 120

Zimbardo, P., x, 133-138

Growing Younger

About the Authors

Robert Morgan Ph.D.

California Psychology License PSY3869
305 Mission Serra Terrace, Chico, CA 95926
Guam Psychology License CP17
Telephone: (530) 892-2131 or (650) 493-4430 ext.. 49
Hawaii Psychology License 632
Fax: (815) 550-4456
Email: rmorgan@itp.edu or morganfoundation@earthlink.net
Rev. 1/21/04

Robert Morgan is Professor and Chair of the Ph.D. Program at the Institute of Transpersonal Psychology in Palo Alto. He is a Fellow of the American Psychological Association (Divisions 12 Clinical, 29 Psychotherapy, 52 International) and the Western Psychological Association. Since 1982 he has served on the Executive Committee & Board of the International Association of Applied Psychologists. He is a member of the International Council of Psychologists, the psychology associations of Guam and California, and the American Counseling Association. He has been listed in the National Register of Mental Health Providers in Psychology since its inception in 1975.

Dr. Morgan completed his psychology doctorate at Michigan State University as Fellow of the National Institute of Mental Health. During this time he had also served as City Human Relations Commissioner. Following postdoctoral work at Hawaii State Hospital, including the founding of its first inpatient therapeutic community adolescent program, he served on the university faculties of Saint Bonaventure University, Nova Scotia's Acadia University, the University of Southern Colorado (USC), San Diego State University, Wilfrid Laurier University, Montana State University, Howard University (Washington, D.C.), San Francisco State University, University of Guam, and free-standing professional schools of psychology since their inception three decades ago.

In addition to chairing departments of Psychology at USC, MSU, and WLU, he was for many years the Dean of Faculty and then Campus Dean at CSPP-SF. He has also served on the Executive Council of CSPP's Board (Faculty Elected Director) as Treasurer, and as Vice President of CSPP's California Community Services, Inc. Subsequently, he was founding President of the USC-affiliated Southern Colorado Community Services, Inc. From 1982-1986, he was Professor of Psychology and Dean for Academic Affairs at the California School of Professional Psychology's Fresno Campus. From 1986-1990, he was professor of Psychology and Academic Vice President at the Pacific Graduate School of Psychology, Palo Alto, and then Professor of Psychology and Department Chair at Montana State University, Billings (1991-1993). From 1994-1996 he was Professor of Psychology and Director of the Psychology Doctoral Program at the California Institute of Integral Studies, San Francisco; from 1997-1999 Professor of Psychology and Program Director at the American School of Professional Psychology, California Campus; 1999-2002 Professor & University of Guam College of Education Graduate Faculty, joining ITP in 2002.

Since 1965, Dr. Morgan has provided clinical and supervisory services to community mental health in California, Canada, Colorado, Guam, Hawaii, Nevada, New York, and North Carolina. Professional consultation over the last four decades has included government agencies from Peace Corps to the U.S. Office of Education, community organizational change groups such as Dr. Martin Luther King Jr.'s SCLC, and the Native American Health Center in Oakland. His current practice includes services to individuals and practitioners, as well as organizational/educational consultation on clinical/ counseling education & training, accreditation and program development. He is President of the Board of Directors, Institute for Community Health Outreach, San Francisco.

While on leave from USC in 1977, he accepted a two-year post with the State of Nevada as Chief, Human Services Education. Here he organized and coordinated statewide mental health manpower, training, research, prevention, legislation, and university education liaison, and represented Nevada on the Advisory Council for the Western Center for Continuing Education in Mental Health of the

Western Interstate Commission in Higher Education (WICHE), a coordinating and advisory body for university education in the 13 western states. He is Founding President of the Division of Applied Gerontology, International Association of Applied Psychology; past Chair and CSPA Board of Directors Representative for the California Psychological Association's Division of Education and Training from 1986-1989 and the CPA Mandatory Continuing Education Psychology Committee (MCEP) 1998-1999. He was on the Scientific Program Committee of the American Psychological Association (APA) for the 1998 World Congress of Psychology in San Francisco and Liaison for the 2002 World Congress in Singapore. In 2001 he received the Distinguished International Psychologist Award from APA's International Psychology Division (52), and was elected liaison to APA's Council of Representatives as President of the Guam Psychological Association 2001-2002.

More than 70 articles, chapters, books, and tests include counseling education, international psychology, applied gerontology, life-span development, clinical/community psychology, social & general-experimental psychology, evaluation, special education, applied transpersonal psychology, the psychology of time, prevention of iatrogenic practice, and graduate education/training in psychology.

Other Books From Morgan Foundation Publishers

TITLES OF BOOKS NOW AVAILABLE:

ELECTROSHOCK: THE CASE AGAINST
Robert F. Morgan, editor
(with Peter Breggin, Leonard Frank, John Friedberg, Bertram Karon, Berton Roueche)
ISBN 1885679025
$25 paperback; subject: health/electroconvulsive

GROWING YOUNGER: MEASURE & CHANGE YOUR BODY'S AGE
Robert F. Morgan & Jane Wilson
ISBN 1885679092
$33 paperback; subject: health/aging

THE IATROGENICS HANDBOOK: A CRITICAL LOOK AT RESEARCH & PRACTICE IN THE HELPING PROFESSIONS.
Robert F. Morgan, editor
(26 professionals for 29 chapters)
ISBN 1885679114
$13 paperback; subject: health/iatrogenic

TRAINING THE TIME SENSE: HYPNOTIC & CONDITIONING APPROACHES
Robert F. Morgan, editor
(with Linn Cooper, Elizabeth Erickson, Milton Erickson, Gary Marshall, Christine Maslach, Paul Sacerdote, Philip Zimbardo)
ISBN 1885679106
$38 paperback; subject: hypnosis/time

UNFORTUNATE BABY NAMES: SLATTERY'S COMPLETE COLLECTION.
THE MOST NOTABLE THOUSANDS FOR DRAMATIC OR OTHER USAGE.
Uncas Slattery
ISBN 1885679084
$28 paperback; subject: humor/reference/baby/theater

Prepaid bookseller price includes postage & charges.
Author, subject, EAN bar code on every book.

Morgan Foundation Publishers
305 Mission Serra Terrace, Chico, CA 95926 USA
Fax (815) 550-4456 Phone (530) 892-2131
email: morganfoundtion@earthlink.net
Web page: http://www.morganfoundationpublishers.com